Core St_____umm____ Cheat Sheet

Finding Neutral Spine

When you hear the term *neutral spine* used in exercises, I'm referring to the neutral position of your spine. You will need to use neutral spine with all core exercises and any other workout that involves lying on the floor.

To keep your back from arching and to practice neutral spine, try this exercise in front of a mirror:

1. **Stand facing the side as you look into a mirror.**

2. **Imagine a ruler extending down along your back from the top of your shoulders or shoulder blades to the bottom of your pelvis or hips.**

   You should be standing tall and straight with everything stacked up neatly as follows: head, shoulders, rib cage, pelvis, and legs.

You can also try this exercise by lying on the floor:

1. **Lie on the floor with your back pressed down.**

   If your back is flat, you shouldn't be able to put your hand between the floor and your back.

2. **Exhale as you bring your knees to your chest and think about the placement of your back on the floor.**

3. **Hold your knees to your chest for a few moments, and then release your legs back to the floor.**

   Can you feel the neutral position of your body as it relaxes on the floor but is actively pressed downward? If so, you should now be able to slip your hand under your lower back and feel the natural curve of your spine, otherwise known as maintaining neutral spine.

Post-Workout Stretches

In Chapter 14 you'll find an energizing series of stretches that you can do after your core workout. As a quick reference, I've listed them below.

- Back extension
- Step back and reach
- Side reach
- Lying spinal rotation
- Spinal rotation

For Dummies: Bestselling Book Series for Beginners

Core Strength For Dummies®

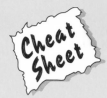

Cheat Sheet

Core Exercise Tips

For the safest and most effective workout, follow these simple and easy tips for *all* core workouts:

- **Use a smooth and steady motion for each exercise.** Never jerk or bounce with any of your movements.

- **Breathe freely while exercising.** Never hold your breath while working out. Breathing freely helps you gain better control of your movements.

- **Remember to stay within your own limits.** Never try an exercise that may risk you hurting yourself or pulling a muscle.

- **If you feel any kind of pain — especially in your joints — never continue the exercise.** Remember that a sharp pain is different from the slight pain or fatigue that you feel in your muscles when you're "going for the burn."

- **Perform the exercises in this book only in the ways in which they're demonstrated.** Adding your own little twist to proven and effective exercises can cause injury. Stick within the guidelines for each exercise, and you'll be fit to the core in no time!

- **Stay within your training range.** When you're just beginning, staying within your own level of comfort and not lifting too heavy a load keeps you from getting an injury and hindering your progress. If you're consistent with your exercise program, you'll see results in a few short weeks.

- **If you feel dizzy or short of breath, stop the exercise.** If you experience dizziness or shortness of breath, stop immediately and breathe deeply while you rest.

- **Exercise in an open space.** Never exercise in a confined or limited space.

- **Always consult your doctor to make sure that you're in good physical shape before you begin a new exercise program.** In addition, if you have a history of back or neck problems or are pregnant, discuss these issues with your healthcare provider to find out if he or she feels that core training is a good choice for you.

- **Warm up properly.** Remember to always warm up properly to get your body ready for exercising and to avoid injury.

- **Cool down properly.** When you're finished working out, cool down and stretch to avoid soreness.

My Top Five Core Exercises

Here it is! My list of the best core strengtheners to help build a better core and a stronger back:

- Abdominal crunch (Chapter 5)
- Bicycle (Chapter 6)
- Plank (Chapter 8)
- Crunches with weights (Chapter 10)
- Legs straight up crunches (Chapter 6)

For Dummies: Bestselling Book Series for Beginners

Core Strength FOR DUMMIES®

by LaReine Chabut

WILEY

Wiley Publishing, Inc.

Core Strength For Dummies®

Published by
Wiley Publishing, Inc.
111 River St.
Hoboken, NJ 07030-5774

www.wiley.com

WILEY

About the Author

LaReine Chabut is a fitness and lifestyle expert, model, and mom, as well as the author of *Exercise Balls For Dummies* (Wiley), *Lose That Baby Fat!* (M.Evans) and *Stretching For Dummies* (Wiley). LaReine is a leading contributing fitness expert for *Shape* and *Fit Pregnancy* magazines and is most recognized as the lead instructor for America's number one exercise video series *The Firm* (with more than three million copies sold worldwide). She has graced the covers of such high-profile magazines as *Shape, Health, New Body,* and *Runner's World,* and has recently appeared on *Dr. Phil, Chelsea Lately* on *E!, CNN, ABC, FOX News, EXTRA, Access Hollywood, Good Day LA,* and *KABC.*

LaReine and her *Lose That Baby Fat* programs can be found at www.pod fitness.com/lareinechabut, where she is a premier trainer for iPods, along with Kathy Smith, David Kirsch, and other top trainers in their field.

As an actress, LaReine penned a sitcom with Meg Ryan entitled *Below the Radar* for the Fox Network and Castle Rock Entertainment. She has co-written and starred in two short films: *Separation Anxiety,* which broadcast on Lifetime Television, and *Good Jill Hunting,* which aired on the Sundance Channel. Her series regular and guest-starring appearances include *Dr. Phil, Chelsea Lately, Linc's, Nash Bridges, The Secret World of Alex Mack, USA High, The Single Guy, Strange Luck, Murder She Wrote,* and *Quantum Leap,* to name a few.

To read more about LaReine, log on to her Web site at www.lareine chabut.com or www.losethatbabyfat.com.

Dedication

This book is dedicated with lots of love to my daughters, Bella and Sofia, who compete for my attention every time I sit down at my desk to write! I do love you both so much . . . and of course to the readers who make it all worth it and buy my books. I thank you all!

Author's Acknowledgments

Writing a book requires a lot of teamwork and, again, I have to thank Rob Dyer at Wiley for encouraging me to write my first book. Who would ever guess that this would be my fourth? Thanks, Rob!

I'd also like to thank the entire staff at Wiley, including Jennifer Connolly, my project editor, who was just great to work with and a busy mom like myself (I could tell by the noise in the background, she started working from home!). Lindsay Lefevere, acquisitions editor, really is good at what she does and was always there for me when I needed her. Krista Hansing, my copy editor, who made everything look nice and consistent and encouraged me to use spell check! My agent at ICM, Andrea Barvzi, to be able to convince me to write a book in a few months! And photographer Nick Horne sat on an exercise ball as he shot the photos and still managed to make me look good. Make-up artist Mina Kang made me look really tan, which is always nice. And last, but certainly not least, Linda Shelton was on my first cover shoot for Shape magazine and served as director for this shoot — thanks, Linda, you really are the best!!

Special thanks to all the models who look so hot! Robert Check is shirtless in all the pictures in this book, and when you see him, you'll know why (thanks to his agent, David Levine, for bringing him to my attention:). Chris Gann took time off from shooting a film to do the shots in Chapters 8 and 10 and filled in as my senior model. And, of course, my beautiful daughter, Bella, and her friend Elizabeth Bartle-Steere did the kids' exercises for me. Last but certainly not least, baby Sofia Gallachi was the best baby I've ever worked with — and never made a peep!

Publisher's Acknowledgments

We're proud of this book; please send us your comments through our Dummies online registration form located at www.dummies.com/register/.

Some of the people who helped bring this book to market include the following:

Acquisitions, Editorial, and Media Development

Project Editor: Jennifer Connolly

Acquisitions Editor: Lynsey Lefevere

Copy Editor: Krista Hansing

Technical Editor: Damon Faust

Senior Editorial Manager: Jennifer Ehrlich

Editorial Supervisor: Carmen Krikorian

Editorial Assistants: Erin Calligan Mooney, Joe Niesen, Jennette ElNagger, and David Lutton

Cartoons: Rich Tennant (www.the5thwave.com)

Cover Photo Credit: Nick Horne

Composition Services

Project Coordinator: Lindsay Stanford

Layout and Graphics: Stacie Brooks, Reuben W. Davis, Sarah Philippart, Christine Williams

Proofreaders: Jessica Kramer, Christine Sabooni

Indexer: Ty Koontz

Publishing and Editorial for Consumer Dummies

    Diane Graves Steele, Vice President and Publisher, Consumer Dummies

    Joyce Pepple, Acquisitions Director, Consumer Dummies

    Kristin A. Cocks, Product Development Director, Consumer Dummies

    Michael Spring, Vice President and Publisher, Travel

    Kelly Regan, Editorial Director, Travel

Publishing for Technology Dummies

    Andy Cummings, Vice President and Publisher, Dummies Technology/General User

Composition Services

    Gerry Fahey, Vice President of Production Services

    Debbie Stailey, Director of Composition Services

Contents at a Glance

Table of Contents

Introduction

• •

Core training is a hot topic these days, isn't it? Just take a look at any magazine or DVD — they all seem to be targeting your core. Yes, having a strong core not only prevents injuries, but it also makes the movements you make on a daily basis easier to manage. So what is core strength and how do you get it? Well, I think it is best described as having fat-free abs and a strong back. I describe the *core* itself as the "bridge" that connects your upper and lower body. So if you have a weak bridge, all your movements will suffer because nothing will make it across that bridge.

Some people call it core training because you're doing just that — increasing the strength in your midsection as you're whittling your waist and developing strong back muscles. Just think of how often you call upon your core to perform movements throughout the day: getting up from your couch or a chair, picking up your children or grandchildren, and sitting at your desk while you're working. All these activities require great core strength — otherwise, you'd walk around hunched over with weak back muscles all day long. Sound familiar? I hope not! I want to show you how to obtain a stronger core with this book and help you gain a better understanding of why it's so important to have a strong core in the first place!

About This Book

This book introduces you to various core exercises that everybody can do — no matter what your age or lifestyle. In fact, there's a chapter for everybody in this book — from kids to seniors — that can help you develop a regular core-training routine to do every day or just learn a few new moves to keep you feeling great! I've included Pilates and yoga workouts, children's exercises, senior exercises, workouts for new moms and babies, weight training for your core, and more. You'll also discover how to stave off workout boredom by adding a few new props, such as the exercise ball and dumbbells. In addition, I cover simple core strengtheners you can do using household objects or the resistance of your own body weight.

This book contains comprehensive sections on special circumstances, like exercising during pregnancy and relieving back pain by targeting your abdominals. I even include a total core workout you can do when you have enough time and aren't rushed to work out. Whatever your interest or age, you're sure to get a good core workout and have some fun doing it!

In this book, I tell you everything you need to know about core training, such as answers to the following questions:

- What muscles am I targeting when I'm strengthening my core?
- What kind of changes can I expect to see in my body from core training?
- How many days a week should I do these core workouts?
- Is it safe to exercise during pregnancy?
- What are the best core strengtheners I can do for back pain?
- Can kids strengthen their core, too?
- Can I stretch out my core?
- Is it safe for senior citizens to exercise?
- Are there core exercises I can do on the exercise ball?
- Will the core workouts be a challenging enough for me if I'm already in shape?

In addition, this book, like all *For Dummies* books, has a friendly and approachable tone that assumes you don't know a whole lot about the subject you're reading — not that you're an actual dummy! It's also important to tell you that like all For Dummies books, you don't have to read it cover to cover . . . instead just flip to the section that best describes you or read a little intro first before moving onto whatever interests you. This book is also useful for learning new core-training techniques for those who already know what they're doing. You can always pick up new techniques from a *For Dummies* book!

Conventions Used in This Book

The focus of this book is on core strengthening in many different situations, while emphasizing safety and proper body alignment. Reading the step-by-step instructions that accompany the photos before you start any of the exercises makes trying these core moves a lot easier and helps to keep your workouts safe and effective.

Check out these conventions I used to make navigating the information in this book a lot easier:

- Most of the core exercise photos show two stages — labeled A and B — demonstrating the beginning and end for each pose.

✔ I use *italics* to point out any new terms or bits of jargon you should know.

✔ Web sites and e-mail addresses appear in `monofont` to help them stand out.

✔ The numbered sets of instructions for the core exercises and the key-words in lists appear in **boldface.**

What You're Not to Read

Although I feel that all the information in this book is important, the sidebars that appear in the gray boxes don't contain information that you absolutely need to know to get a good core workout. However, these sidebars do contain great tips and information about your health, so I encourage you to read them at some point.

Foolish Assumptions

As I mentioned earlier in the introduction, this book is for people who don't have a lot of prior knowledge about the subject at hand (in this case, core training and your current level of fitness). Keeping this goal in mind, I made a few assumptions about you, the reader:

✔ You're interested in core strengthening and want to make it part of your life.

✔ You don't have much experience with core exercises and want to know more.

✔ You're ready, willing, and able to find out more about core training and how to do the exercises in this book.

If this sounds like you, then you've come to the right place!

How This Book Is Organized

Core Strength For Dummies is divided into six different parts, each one with a unique focus. You can go directly to whichever part interests you the most or start at the beginning to gather some information and a checklist of what you'll need to know before you begin each core-strengthening chapter. Following are the parts and what you can find in them.

Part I: Core Basics

If you're new to core training, reading Part I is the way to go. Part I covers all the important issues you want to know *before* you begin your core program.

Part I covers these topics:

- ✔ Who should exercise their core
- ✔ How often you should be working your core
- ✔ How you can reshape your core
- ✔ Props you can use to enhance core exercises
- ✔ The benefits of a strong core

Part II: Core Workouts to Help You Sculpt Your Trouble Areas

Part II is organized in a very logical manner — Chapter 5 starts off with a series of beginning exercises, and then the chapters progress with core exercises that are illustrated for various individual body parts. Finally, Chapter 8 finishes with a total body workout to strengthen your entire body.

Because I believe you should work out in a progressive manner (starting with the simplest exercises first), I strongly encourage starting with the beginner exercises in Chapter 5 and then progressing through the chapters until you reach Chapter 8. These chapters concentrate first on the abdominals and then on the butt; finally, you put it all together for a total body workout focusing on your core.

Part III: Developing Core Strength Using Accessories

Part III shows you a variety of core exercises you can do while using accessories. This section may be the most useful part of the book for you if you already have knowledge of core training and want to beat boredom by adding a few new techniques or a few new moves.

In Chapter 9, I show you core exercises using an exercise ball and offer you a ball chart so you know how to pick the right size of ball. Chapter 10 contains core exercises using dumbbells that you can add to any workout you already have or just use alone for core strengthening.

This part ends with nice primer on ab machines that you can use at your gym to get a nice six-pack!

Part IV: Adding Variety to Your Core Routine

Part IV is a fantastic section on recruiting different training techniques to help with core strengthening. If you've ever wanted to try Pilates, Chapter 11 is the one for you. This chapter contains photo illustrations of Pilates strengthening exercises that help you get a killer core.

Chapter 12 is a chapter for anyone interested in yoga — and you'll love doing the poses! Whether you're a beginner or you know all about the sun salutation, you'll like trying these poses that place a special emphasis on your core.

Part IV also contains Chapter 14, for stretching your core. It shows some fun and practical stretches for the abs, hips, and back that'll help keep you strong and flexible for years to come.

Part V: Special Situations

No matter what stage of life you're in, core exercises can improve your *daily* life. Check out Chapter 15 for pregnancy and postnatal core exercises that help you to relax and strenghten your body before and after you have your baby. Get the kids together to perform a series of fun exercises that Chapter 16 provides, which help your kids build basic core strength and learn the skills needed to stay fit for a lifetime. And finally, Chapter 18 contains core exercises that address the needs of anyone over the age of 60. If you're in one of these demographics, this part has something for you!

Part VI: The Part of Tens

In every *For Dummies* book, you find The Part of Tens. The last three chapters in this book contain top-ten lists of fun facts about the different things you'll get from core training and what you can use to enhance your workout at home.

Chapter 19 lists ten best ways to train your core, while in Chapter 20, I offer ten dietary changes you can make to whittle your core and get fat free abs. Finally, Chapter 21 offers ten different items you can use in your house to make core strengthening fast and fun!

Icons Used in This Book

In this book, you'll find different pictures in the margins, or *icons,* that give you useful information along the way. Reading these icons before you try the actual exercises is helpful because many of them suggest easier or better ways of performing each one.

Here's a list of icons used in this book:

The Tip icon gives you useful information that'll make your life easier as it relates to core training. I may point you to a specific chapter or resource, or provide hints to modify an exercise or to make it easier. For instance, a Tip icon may tell you how to breathe during an exercise to keep you from holding your breath, or it may tell you to maintain a neutral spine.

As you may have guessed, this icon points out really important information that you need to keep in mind. Very valuable information comes with these icons, so don't skip 'em!

The Warning icon highlights information that keeps you from hurting yourself. Read the information listed under this icon before you attempt each exercise. You'll be glad you did!

Where to Go from Here

Core Strength For Dummies is a reference guide for beginners and an introduction to performing core-strengthening exercises. You can start reading at the very beginning of this book to gather a little information first, or you can dive right in and tear out the yellow Cheat Sheet in the front of this book to take with you as you're running out the door to a core class.

If you're not sure where you want to start, I suggest browsing the table of contents to get a sense of exactly what this book covers and what topics interest you. You may find that you already know the basics but have always wanted to know how to use an exercise ball, so you can immediately flip to that chapter.

If you fall into one of the special circumstances groups, you may want to go directly to that section to find which chapter covers your special needs. If you're like me, you may just want to go directly to the workout chapters that pertain to you and learn some new moves.

And if you know all about core training already and just want to brush up on your exercises a bit, you can turn to the index to find out which information pertains to you.

Wherever you choose to start, it's great that you're here. Enjoy!

Part I
Core Basics

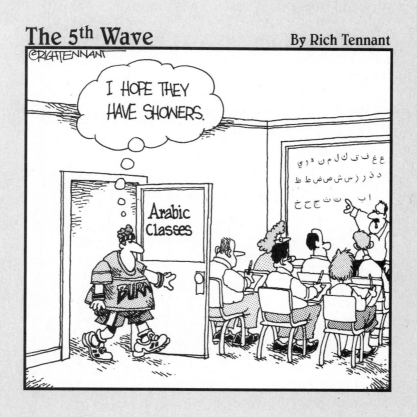

In this part . . .

1know that you know a strong core is good for you, but in Chapter 1, I cover *why* having a strong core is actually good for you. I also answer all the questions you may have about your core — like where it is located, why you need to strengthen it, and how to acquire core strength through specific exercises.

In Chapter 2, I get into the anatomy of your core a little bit, which will give you a better understanding of what muscles you're working and which one's you aren't. I show you how to evaluate your core stability and test your present level of fitness so you'll have a starting point for your new core-training program. I even help you understand what you can do to reshape your core to the best of your ability — with a little help from me.

Chapter 3 includes everything you need to know to get started, including what props you might want to use and how much space you'll need. I also give you the basics of a safe core-training program, including guidelines for beginners and advanced exercisers.

I wrap it all up in Chapter 4, where I show you a few warm-ups to increase your core temperature and prepare your body for core training.

Chapter 1

Finding Your Core Strength

- -

In This Chapter

▶ Discovering the benefits of core training

▶ Getting answers to all your questions about core strength

▶ Exploring different techniques used for core training

▶ Discovering new sports that need core strengthening

▶ Developing core strength for relaxation

▶ Finding fun ways to incorporate core training

▶ Adding accessories to your core workout

- -

*W*hether you're looking to nix your muffin top (the fat that hangs over the top of your belt!) or get washboard abs (better known as a six-pack), core training is a powerful tool that requires great strength in your abdominal muscles and back. The results can certainly be just like magic — killer abs and a long, straight spine; new ease of everyday movements; increased ability for all your muscles to work together; and a sense of really being fit to the core.

Of course, I'm aware that many of you may want to just tone up your tummy and think it takes only a few days of eating less (and you know who you are); others of you may be wrought with fear and dread that you'll be forced to do a hundred sit-ups! Well, just as in everyday life, the truth lies somewhere in the middle.

Believe it or not, the ideas and techniques I use in this book were never part of a Marines-style workout and were never used in a torture chamber, but you may see some of my moves in a real gym where boxers train or many athletes go to work out. I like to get a little *old school* because *I know* that many of you (me included) have become soft around the middle from watching way too many reality shows and eating a little too much pizza. So read on to get a tighter, toner tummy and stronger back, which will help you zip up those pants or wear that bikini you've been stashing in the back of your drawer. Isn't it time?

First Things First: Locating Your Core

This is it, the phenomenon on which this entire book is based: the miraculous capability of our bodies to grow in strength and tap into the amazing power located in the abs and back, or core. Before we can use this amazing power, we need to understand how it works, how to strengthen it, and how to maintain it.

When you hear people talking about "the core," they're actually referring to the muscles that lie deep within the abs and back. Some of these muscles include the transversus abdominal, the muscles of the pelvic floor, and the waist muscles or obliques. These muscles are where all your core movements originate and are the main source of stability in your body to maintain an upright standing position. Whether picking up your baby or toddler, carrying groceries or boxes, or walking, these core muscles help keep your body stable and balanced.

With this new focus on the importance of core strength, the entire fitness industry has moved toward training the body as a whole instead of focusing on separate muscle groups (see Chapter 14). Incorporating core training into every workout you do has been proven to provide exceptional benefits to your entire body that you need to stay injury free for life (see the section "Benefits to Core Training" for more on the benefits core training produces for your body). You can enhance this type of functional training for your core with anything that challenges your balance, like the exercise ball (see Chapter 9) and wobble boards.

The Five W's of Core Training

Using a "just the facts" approach, I've gathered the following information to make up the five W's — the who, what, where, when and why's of core training. Read on to find out the answers to your burning questions before you embark on your core training.

Who needs core training?

Everyone needs core training! As I mention throughout this book, core strengthening is vital to your health — not just for physical appearances — because the core serves as the "bridge" that connects your upper body with your lower body. All of your movements suffer if you don't have a strong connection between your upper and lower body. And all internal organs cannot be supported without having the strength of your internal and external girdle, known as the core. Training only your upper body and leaving your core susceptible to weakness creates a muscle imbalance, which leads to injury. You need to have a strong midsection to provide your body with the strength it needs to walk up stairs, pick up children, bend down to pick something up, or reach for something high on a shelf. No one is exempt from needing a strong core — not even at tax time!

What can I do to acquire core strength?

You can do many things to acquire core strength, all of which are in this book! You can vary the intensity of the many exercises in each chapter simply by adding more repetitions and increasing the number of sets you do.

And by some stroke of genius, walking is the number one form of core strengthening that *anyone* can do at every stage in life. Walking calls upon the internal abdominal muscles and your back muscles to facilitate each step you take, which creates a stronger corset or core. Hiking is effective also because you have the added resistance of a varied terrain as you walk up and down hills. And you can also try running, which helps speed up weight loss and lose that layer of fat that is inevitably covering up your washboard abs.

Where is the best place to work out to get a stronger core?

At home! If you have to go to a gym or go outdoors, either bad weather will intervene or you'll probably find some excuse to not make it out the door. Believe me, I've heard them all . . . and that's why I've designed the exercises in this book to be done right at home (or at the gym, or anywhere else, for that matter!) so you have no excuse not to work out. The exercises in each chapter take up very little space — and you will even find a chapter on ten household items you can use to help train your core (see Chapter 21).

When should I do core training?

Any time of day is fine, as long as your muscles are warm. A lot of trainers will tell you to work out first thing in the morning, at the end of the day, or both. And a lot of good research exists to support such recommendations. But as far as I'm concerned, whatever works for you is best. If this statement sounds a little obvious, then get ready, here comes another one: It's better to do it than not do it. I mean that if you try to force yourself into a schedule that doesn't really work for you, you probably won't stick with your new core-training program. Find a time of day that's convenient for you, and make that your special time for yourself.

Consistency is the key!

Why should I strengthen my core?

You should strengthen your core to make all your movements effortless and keep your body injury free. And if that's not enough motivation, you should embark on core training so you can zip up your jeans or wear a belt around your waist. That's enough motivation for anyone; I don't care who you are . . . or when you had your baby! Fitting into those skinny jeans requires one key element: losing weight in your waist. And you can't do that without core exercises.

The How's of Core Strengthening

You may be wondering how you're going to set your core-training plan into action. Following the exercises in this book is the first step and, lucky for you, I've also included the following, commonly asked "how" questions, which give you all the answers you need to get the job done.

How often should I exercise to strengthen my core?

To increase core strength in your abs and back muscles, the general rule is to do strengthening exercises at least three to five times a week. Elite athletes will obviously exercise more than that — two or even three times a day. But let's be realistic. For those of us who are not getting *paid* to exercise and be in peak condition, it's pretty difficult to find the time to work out that much. If you're looking to increase your present level of fitness, I recommend that you engage in focused core exercises every other day. When you have reached your goal of toning your midsection and strengthening your back, I'm confident that you can maintain your new physique by doing the core exercises contained in this book three times a week.

How long should I exercise each time I work out my core?

You're going to love this next section, because I tell you that less is more! Studies have demonstrated that the optimum effectiveness of an exercise is reached after your heart rate is elevated for approximately 20 to 30 minutes. Train less, and you don't really give your body time to adapt properly to your new elevated heart rate; train more, and you risk what I call, the burn-out factor. I'm sure you're familiar with this problem: You embark on a new fitness program and go at it so fiercely and competitively that after a few weeks, you either have an injury or get really run down and have to take some time off. Moderation is the key to everything in life, so stick with the 20- to 30-minute rule before you increase the length of your workouts. Remember, slow and steady wins the race!

How intense should the exercise feel?

When it comes to working out your core, the old cliché "no pain, no gain" is definitely wrong. In fact, pain is the most precise indicator of an exercise that has gone too far, either in degree or in duration. If you're exercising to the point that your muscles sizzle inside or are quivering, or you find that you are becoming less able to hold the position you are doing, back off. A core exercise should feel no more than slightly uncomfortable. When you reach the point of resistance in your abdominals, stay there and hold it for a moment before relaxing and taking a few breaths. You'll find that you can increase your repetitions after a while or perhaps in a few days; if you force the issue, though, it'll only set you back further than you were when you started. Keep the following ideas in mind when gauging the intensity of your exercising:

- **You should feel slight exertion in the muscle that you are exercising.** This tension should definitely not cross the line to pain or discomfort. The rest of your body should be in a position that is relaxed and totally tension free. If your body feels awkward or tense, modify the exercise by using a prop such as an exercise ball or pair of hand weights to help you focus on the intended muscle. Remember, exercise should be a positive experience, not a form of self-torture.

- **You should feel the exertion of the exercise only in the intended muscle, never in a joint.** Pain in your joints signals irritation in the joint, so you definitely want to let up if that happens. Conversely, you should not feel tension or tightness in any other part of your body. If you do, as

I mentioned before, ease up on the exercise or try using props like an exercise ball to modify the exercise. Throughout this book, I give you several different ways to do an abdominal crunch; if one doesn't seem to fit your body, you'll be better off trying one that feels more comfortable.

Should I see a doctor before I begin a core-strengthening program?

Always consult a physician before embarking on any new fitness program, even a seemingly low-impact program such as core training. But it's imperative that you speak to your health-care professional before undertaking a regular core exercise program if you have back problems or an injury that has not healed completely. Your doctor can advise you about specific exercises you can do to focus on or to avoid, and can help customize a core-training program to help meet your unique needs.

Benefits to Core Training

Go ahead — ask your doctor, your trainer, or your physical therapist whether you should do core-strengthening exercises. Get ready to hear the exact same answer from all of them: a resounding *yes*. Even though they don't make a dime giving such advice, why would all these professionals so enthusiastically recommend core training? I give you the skinny in the sections that follow.

Overall benefits

Although the specific benefits of core training vary individually, remember these overall, general benefits that core training provides for everyone:

- ✔ Challenging exercises to help you get in touch with your body and tap into your inner core strength
- ✔ Increased performance in whatever sports you choose to do
- ✔ Injury prevention due to increased strength and stamina
- ✔ Functional exercises that provide additional ease of movements throughout your daily life and activities

Weight (less) benefits

As anyone may guess, having fat around the middle or belly fat has many drawbacks, including great health risks. Core training helps you not only look better, but also increase your health and chances at living a longer, more physically active life. Read on to find more ways core training will give you the preventative medicine you need for a lifetime.

Living longer

The fat that lies in the belly becomes part of your abdomen. As you widen and grow in the midsection, this fat gets stored in the deepest layer of the abdominal wall and disperses in the way of fatty acids into your bloodstream.

The fatty cells accumulate in your liver and, eventually, into your circulation. This build-up of fat cells can lead to type 2 diabetes, high cholesterol, and heart disease. The belly fat then becomes resistant to dieting and needs the help of targeted core training to whittle and tone the area. So besides getting a smaller waist, with core training, you'll be saving your life!

Lowering blood pressure

Unfortunately, the risk of high blood pressure (better known as hypertension) increases with age. However, you don't need to sit back and wait for hypertension or high blood pressure to strike. And that's why you're reading this book, right? Regular exercise can help prevent high blood pressure, which, in turn, reduces the risk of cardiovascular disease and even stroke. If your blood pressure is already high, regular exercise can help you control it for good.

Physical activity and exercise make your heart stronger, and thus able to pump more blood easier and with less effort. So the less your heart has to work, the less pressure or force is exerted on your arteries.

Interestingly, exercise can lower your blood pressure the same way some blood pressure medications can. And that should be enough to get you off the couch and going! Once you do, it takes approximately three months of regular exercise to have an impact or stabilize your blood pressure. And as long as you stick with exercise, the benefit of lowering your blood pressure will last a lifetime!

Lowering your risk of developing type 2 diabetes

Previously in this chapter, I talked about belly fat and how it affects the internal organs of your body — and just how resistant it becomes to dieting without exercise to "shake it up." Yes, there is a correlation between diabetes and the location of fat in the body. People with a heavier deposit of fat around the hips and thighs have a higher risk for insulin resistance, high cholesterol, and high blood pressure.

Exercise, especially cardio and targeted core workouts, improves blood cholesterol. And you get this benefit from exercise even if you don't lose any weight! Three months of regular exercise is the recommended guideline for lowering triglyceride levels in people with type 2 diabetes and increasing good cholesterol levels, or HDL. And the added bonus you get from exercising to control or lower your type 2 diabetes is that even your blood pressure returns to a better level.

Countering bone loss with exercise

Bone loss, or osteoporosis, is a real disease that affects men and women. It is especially prevalent in postmenopausal women because estrogen levels, which protect bones, drop after menopause. When bones become brittle, they weaken and put you at a greater risk of fracture.

Exercise of the right type, or weight-bearing exercises (see Chapter 10), helps keep bones strong by stimulating new bone cells to multiply and produce more bone. If you don't like using dumbbells and weights, you can use the resistance of your own body weight, as I show in Chapter 13 with a series of push-ups and dips.

You can also use the weight of your own body to counter bone loss with cardio exercise like jogging, running, or, my fave of all time, jumping rope (see the skipping rope exercise in Chapter 4). The force you use to push each foot to the ground during "high-impact" cardio exercise helps build up muscle and strengthens the bones in your body. Stronger bones lead to fewer injuries because, when you fall, you don't risk a fracture if your bones are strong — just one more great reason to get up and get going.

Added physical and mental bonuses

I'm sure you already know, but I do like to motivate with a reminder that exercise benefits your body and mind, and helps improve your level of fitness. Weight-bearing exercise is best for strengthening bones. In the following sections, consider more examples of what core strengthening can specifically add to your game.

Better posture

Tall and erect posture not only makes you look leaner; it is also essential to allow your body to perform the way it was meant to. What's more, good posture aids dramatically in facilitating free and effective breathing. The main enemy of good posture, however, is a weak lower back and slackened abs.

Core training can help you correct muscular imbalances that lead to incorrect skeletal alignment. One cause of this kind of imbalance is using one side of your body more than the other, like when you carry your toddler on the same side, or always carry your briefcase in the same hand, or perhaps even wear your shoulder bag on the same shoulder. Such chronic imbalances can rob you of energy and efficiency from movement, or even result in back pain. Regular core strengthening can help balance out these bad habits, so you'll be sure to stand up straight.

Increased range of motion

Over time, muscles naturally tend to shorten and become tight. So as you age, your ability to fully utilize movement in your body becomes compromised. Strengthening the core of the body can help dramatically increase the range of motion in your joints, which not only enhances your performance in any chosen sport, but also helps in your everyday life by making it possible for you to reach higher or lower, bend farther, and reduce nagging aches and pains from weak muscles. You'll gain an increased ability to function on a daily basis from having core strength — and you'll also be able to tighten your belt!

Injury prevention

Numerous studies attest to the fact that core-strengthening exercises enable you not only to decrease the severity of injuries and the time it takes to recover from an injury, but also to reduce the chance of being injured in the first place. Core training has also been proven to reduce back pain when you accidentally overuse your muscles when engaging in sports. In short, although nothing can prevent injury completely, having a strong core can be a very low-cost, long-term insurance policy for your body, whether you engage in sports or not.

Stress reduction

Stress is a part of life! Some stress (a little) is even good and can help spur you on to take action and achieve great things. But too much stress can actually threaten your health and well-being. Although you can take advantage of several ways of coping with stress, remember that exercise can be therapeutic. Of course, regular workouts can help individual muscles release and relax, but the deep, regular breathing that is so important to exercising can also oxygenate your blood and produce a reduction in overall stress and anxiety.

Regular core training promotes relaxation not only of your body, but also of your mind as you embark on exercises that tap into your inner strength (see Chapter 12 on using yoga poses with core training). Most of you expect that exercise helps individual muscles release tension and relax, but the regular breathing that is so important to effective exercise can also help oxygenate your blood and produce a reduction in overall stress and anxiety. The exercises in a good core-strengthening program can provide an effect like a moving meditation, tapping into energy sources that lie deep within your inner abdominals as you position your body for the next exercise.

Concentrated focus on each area in your core helps you target the muscles you're working. Correct positioning and appropriate exertion that you need to use with the core exercises help block out other stress-inducing thoughts, such as your schedule, your finances, or your kids. In this way, exercise not only strengthens your body, but it expands your mind as well. And the rush you get from those naturally occurring hormones known as endorphins is a self-imposed high you can't beat!

Reduced muscle soreness

For years doctors have thought that the achy feeling you get in your muscles after working out intensely was the result of lactic acid build-up in the tissues of your muscles. Lactic acid is a normal by-product of the process of turning oxygen into energy, also known as *glycolysis*. When you work extra hard, your blood does not carry enough oxygen to wash your muscles clean of lactic acid and a residue builds up. But now cutting-edge thinking attributes this discomfort to tiny tears in muscle fibers caused by the requirements of un-familiar training (also known as *eccentric* movements). By helping to ensure that your muscles are strong and flexible with regular exercise and core training, you can protect yourself from sustaining the microscopic injuries caused by newly intense levels of exercise.

Decreased muscle tension

Strong muscles are one of the major benefits of core strengthening, along with decreased tension in your muscles. What may not be so obvious is the hidden toll persistent muscle tightness can take on you. For one thing, chronically tight muscles can actually choke off their own circulation. This diminished blood flow can result in raised blood pressure, as well as a decrease in oxygen and nutrients in the muscle tissues, which can cause toxic waste products to build up in the cells. The end result is persistent fatigue, as well as aches and pains in your tense muscles.

What's more, if a muscle stays partially contracted for an abnormally long time, the muscle can actually begin to shorten, which not only limits your range of motion, but also can weaken the muscle, create tightness, and make the muscle less effective.

And did you know that muscles that are constantly contracted require more energy to move than a relaxed muscle? As a result, you wind up wasting precious energy with every movement. So in addition to reducing tension in your muscles, a regular exercise and core-strengthening program can actually elevate the level of your overall health. Pretty amazing what preventative medicine exercise really is, isn't it?

Useful and Fun Techniques for Developing Core Strength

You probably agree that choosing the right form of exercise for yourself is very personal. Everyone prefers different flavors of ice cream; it's the same with core training. Although the goal is always the same — to tone and whittle the waist and get a stronger back — you can accomplish that in some new and challenging ways. Here I share some of the ways that I find to be the most fun — and the best ones to help you forget about exercising in the first place!

Yoga

In Chapter 12, you'll find different poses used in the practice of yoga that flow right through your core and challenge your strength! Yoga's not for wimps! And people who think it is should take a class sometime just to see how intense it can be. Because yoga requires great strength to support the entire weight of your body as you hold a plank position seemingly for hours or hold your body straight in the air during a headstand, you will most likely walk away from any yoga class with a new admiration for anyone who practices it. Requiring more flexibility than a stretch class and more stamina than an aerobics class, yoga ranks right up there among my top five ways to get great abdominal strength and a really strong back (better known as your core).

Pilates

Pilates is a great core strengthener because all of its movements originate from your core (see Chapter 11 for Pilates-based core exercises). When Joseph Pilates first came up with his series of Pilates exercises, he created them to rehabilitate injuries of wounded patients during the war. With a system of pulleys and springs, he transformed hospital beds into a contraption used for physical therapy. The terms Pilates "reformer" and Pilate's "bed" were derived from this system.

In Chapter 11, I show a series of "mat" exercises that are used on the reformer or Pilates bed once you've mastered them on the floor. They are all fabulous core strengtheners — fun but challenging to do!

Wii Fit

Wow! New moms are in love with Wii Fit, and so are kids and their parents. And now I know why: It's fun and very hip to do. Wii fit is a video game that helps you build and tone your muscles as you watch and play along on the television. How fun is that? It even helps you lose weight with all kinds of new programs that have you jogging in place and even doing yoga (one of the most popular ones with the ladies).

What Wii Fit really is, however, is just a clever way to get you to work out, disguised as a video game. You can choose from many options if you want to train your core, and you can even enter your individual fitness level. After you do, you're given other menu items to chose from, which makes Wii Fit fun and engaging at the same time. And I know your friends will want to use it once they hear about it, because everyone wants to be in the know when it comes to something new, right?

Of course, the Wii Fit initial sell-out success across the country prompted a lot of press, but the real question is, does it work? If you haven't made it out of the house to the gym or taken a walk lately, it definitely works! In other words, it's better than sitting around thinking about working out, especially for busy moms who don't have time to make it to the gym — it's perfect!

For more information on Nintendo Wii Fit, visit www.nintendo.com/wii.

Training with a partner

If you're anything like me, having someone waiting for you to work out helps because you know you have to show up! And a training partner who encourages you and depends on you is the perfect complement to any workout session. By helping you with your form or counting out your reps, a partner can help you get far more out of your core routine than you may be able to do on your own.

Good, consistent communication is the key to helping each other exercise properly, and so is knowing when someone has been pushed to his limits. Go slow, talk, and listen, and you'll be amazed at the speedy progress you will make. Together you can encourage each other and try new exercises you may not be able to alone (see Chapter 17 for a few fun exercises to help strengthen your core as a pair). Pair up and don't disappoint the person waiting for you — use the buddy system!

Got Skills? Get Core Strength

Okay, here's my roundup of sports that I think are pretty well rounded! Training your core for different sports makes you a better athlete or perhaps just a better weekend warrior.

Check this list to see if doing any of the following sports could enhance your performance with the core-strengthening exercises in this book.

Running and hiking

When you go for a run or a hike, you use the core muscles in your abs and back to move your legs, known as the large muscle groups in the lower half. These muscles need strengthening so they can support all the dynamic movements your body demands as you run with force and place tons of pressure on your lower-back muscles.

I suggest trying the core exercises in Chapter 6 as a perfect complement to any running, hiking, or biking program. Those exercises help you strengthen your abdominals and encourage you to stand tall as you move swiftly along.

Racquet sports

If you play racquet sports, you may notice that you generally use one side of your body — or the dominant arm — more than the other, thus creating an imbalance, or asymmetry, between your two sides. When training for racquet sports, remember to always strengthen both sides equally because an imbalance can lead to injury. I suggest using weights to strength your arms and waist on both sides of your body equally, as I show in Chapter 10. And check out my model with no shirt, while you're at it — he does a lot of core training, and it shows!

Basketball

Basketball is truly a total-body sport that requires some very specific movements to shoot the ball and move with maximum mobility. The core exercises in this book will truly help increase your jump shot, your power, and hopefully your ability to make your free throws (for you, Shaq . . . nobody's perfect!). Try the exercises in Chapter 14 if you're a real basketball player, or even if you just want to whittle your middle and move faster!

Football

Because of the enormous number of collisions that occur regularly in football, a strong and flexible core is essential. Coaches and trainers put a lot of time into making sure their athletes are strong and flexible, to protect them from severe injuries.

However, sometimes you see a football player who seems to concentrate only on being big and not having a six-pack or washboard abs. Big may be good for tackling another person, but you still have to be able to get back up using your abs and back after you get knocked down. Try Chapter 8 if you're at interested in doing that just that; it will test your strength, I guarantee!

Swimming

I don't know about you, but I've never seen a swimmer with an ounce of body fat! In fact, of all the sports I mention, I think swimmers as a group have the best cores of all. Maybe because they're stretched out in the water all day long and forced to use the power of their back and legs to move them through it, or maybe because their lats and waist get defined with every swimming stroke there is. Whatever the case may be, swimmers have strong cores and undoubtedly know the importance of core strength. Swimmers, take note: Strong and toned abs and back muscles go a long way toward increasing your range of motion in your stroke and, therefore, your overall speed.

Skiing

Skiing requires good coordination, balance, and, of course, a strong core to help you move around those large hills of snow! The stronger your back and legs are, the looser you are when you ski, making you more agile so you'll be able to maneuver your skis better.

Soccer

Soccer is all about the lower body and engaging the abs, butt, and back for speed and range of motion. The core gets called upon constantly when kicking the ball and lifting your leg to do so. For every movement in soccer, whether it's running down the field or passing the ball down the field, your core needs to be tight to control all the small and twisting movements that your back needs. See Chapter 7 for some butt and core exercises that will have you playing like . . . what's his name? Oh, yeah, bend it like Beckham!

Cycling

Cyclists are another group that you may never see an ounce of fat on, and that's because cycling combines cardio with core- and lower-body-strengthening exercise. Anyone who's ever ridden a bike for a long time knows how tight your back can get from bending over for long stretches. The power you need to push the pedals also requires great back and abdominal strength.

For some good core strengtheners to increase your distance, I suggest the bicycle crunch in Chapter 5. It not only works your abs better than traditional crunches, but the twisting motion you get when you do a bicycle crunch tones and tightens your waist muscles, too. It's great for making fast turns when cycling!

Gymnastics

Gymnastics requires a strong body, which is evident when you look at any gymnast on television during the Olympics. Strong back, tight abdominals, and a killer tush! All great core assets! As a gymnast springboards or vaults into a pose, you can bet she's using her core muscles to get there. The foundation of every movement a gymnast makes is located in the core. The extremities of the body, the arms and legs, are used only as anchors when the gymnast gets where she's going.

Step aerobics

Your core muscles propel all the fast and furious moves you'll find in an aerobics class. Stepping, pumping, and so on in a step aerobics class require strong butt and lower-back muscles located in your core. These powerhouse muscles work along with the abdominals to help you move effortlessly through step sequences. And just as in gymnastics, the arms and legs serve as anchors to help steady you as you move throughout the movements.

Weight lifting

Any weight-bearing exercise uses your core, or "bridge," of the body to transition all the movements. In fact, any resistance exercise requires you to engage your abdominals to contract as you pick up something or pull it into your body, or push it over your head. If you try doing any of these exercises with weak abdominals, you'll be hunching your shoulders and rounding your back before you know it! Lifting any kind of weight, either body weight or hand weights, requires you to use your core strength. And when you add cardio, you'll start shedding the outside layer of fat over your six-pack or washboard abs. Don't worry, they're there — they just haven't peeked through yet.

Walking

I mentioned before that walking is the number one exercise for strengthening core muscles and losing weight. That's because each step you take uses the same frequent motion that calls upon your butt, hip, back, and abdominal muscles.

Because all the core areas are called upon at the same time to work together, each step increases the potential for weight loss and enhances your core training. Walking is the best form of exercise because you can do it anywhere and at any stage in your life. The only thing that will change is your pace!

Using Exercise Balls to Build Core Strength

The most portable and most popular of all the accessories to help people build or rebuild core strength is still the exercise ball (take a look at *Exercise Balls For Dummies* by yours truly). The exercise ball is unsurpassed for core strengthening, and the exercise ball is the main piece of equipment you'll need. Cost-effective at around $20, it also doesn't require much room in your home. In addition, it is relatively maintenance free, so you won't have to worry about repairing it if it breaks or even about getting a new one, as you would with a treadmill, elliptical trainer, or universal weight machine. Exercise balls are the best for working your core muscles because they provide a lack of stability that requires you to use your abdominal and back muscles to maintain your balance and steady yourself. Because an exercise ball is the easiest piece of equipment to transport, it's ideal if you're traveling and don't want to miss a workout.

In addition, the portability of the core exercises in this book makes these exercises easy to do anywhere and at any time. And if you've decided to use the exercise ball to help you achieve your core-training goals faster, you can find one at the gym for you to use. Check out the following sections to find out the advantages and disadvantages of gym or in-home training so you can pick the right one for you.

Using core exercise balls at the gym

When you walk onto the training floor at your local gym or health center, you'll notice an abundance of balls used for core training. (Many gyms provide group classes for core training and provide a ball for you.)

Gyms that carry balls usually sell them at the retail stores located inside the clubs. At the club retail stores, most balls are already filled with air, which serves two purposes:

✔ You can see the actual size of the ball and try it out.

✔ Professionals can fill the ball with air to its correct diameter.

Keep in mind that, as with anything you'd purchase at a boutique-type store (like a yoga mat), you'll probably pay more for a ball at your local gym unless it comes with some kind of a health club discount.

Using core exercise balls at home

When it comes to joining a gym, membership fees at most gyms seem to be climbing fast — plus you have to commit for a full year. For a lot of people, this cost gives just one more excuse they need to not achieve their fitness goal and put off working out. Even more intimidating is the fact that you can see all different kinds of equipment on the racks and floor at the gym, and need to pay a trainer to just learn how to use them! Sometimes even I get confused finding the differences between all these different machines and pieces of equipment and how I'm supposed to use them.

That's where your home gym comes in! And I'm going to help you build it so you can increase your core strength and put on muscle instead of spending your hard-earned money on a gym membership that you'll never use.

Best core exercises to do with the exercise ball

The following is the best of the best pulled from the chapters in this book. You can use the core-strengthening exercises in this book with your new accessory, and I've included where to find them in each chapter.

Abdominal crunches

The sit-up or ab crunch on the ball (Chapter 9), which has you lying with your lower back on the ball and doing crunches as you normally would, targets the abdominal muscles. Do these slowly for one set of ten repetitions to start, before adding on more sets.

Bridge lifts

The bridge lift in Chapter 9 is an all-over good position to use on the ball for core training. Lie on your back, place the ball under your feet, and slowly lift your hips off the floor. When you've found your balance, try using your butt and hamstring muscles to curl the ball toward your butt and back out again. Perform one set of ten reps.

Squats with ball

Squats! Can't beat them for sore work. In Chapter 13, you'll use the classic squat position, then hold the ball out in front of you at chest level and perform squats. Perform one set of ten reps.

Push-ups with feet on the ball

The push-ups in Chapter 9 call on your abdominals, back, and butt muscles. Place your hands shoulder width apart on the floor and, keeping your stomach muscles tense, perform a standard push-up. These ball push-ups are a lot harder than traditional push-ups, so aim for only one set of ten reps.

Wall squats

To work your abs, hips, and butt, place the ball behind your lower back between you and a wall. Squat slowly, allowing the ball to roll along the wall against your back. Do one set of ten to begin.

You can perform the weight-training exercises in Chapter 13, like the chest press and the overhead press, while sitting on the ball. That way, you get the benefit of working your core and your other body parts at the same time. You use your abdominal muscles to stabilize yourself on the ball — in other words, to keep from falling off! Use lighter weights until you get used to sitting on the ball, and do one set of ten reps for each exercise.

Chapter 2

Reshaping Your Core

• •

In This Chapter

▶ Knowing what muscles are targeted in your core workout

▶ Understanding how having a strong core means gaining a stronger back

▶ Discovering the results you can reap from having a stronger core

▶ Breathing properly using your core muscles

▶ Taking good care of your core

• •

Many health and fitness experts have realized that it's important to strengthen the core muscles along with the other muscles in the body. By strengthening the core, experts have found that it can lessen a lot of health problems concerning posture and other back problems.

So what that means is that a well-conditioned core leads to good posture and increased endurance of the back all day long. That's because muscles that are located in the core are actually the ones that initiate the proper stabilization of the whole upper and lower torso of the body.

For those who wish to know and understand why it is important to strengthen the core muscles, I give you a quick refresher on the muscles located in your core that will be assisting you in your workouts. The pictures of the muscles located in your core contained in this chapter will give you a reference of how they connect your core to the rest of your body.

Rounding Up Your Core Muscles

Swimming, running, and biking all require one thing: good core strength. You can pedal harder, run longer, and swim faster with core training because, as you know by now, a weak core means a weak body. But it's hard to train your core if you're not sure what it is, so in the following sections, I unveil the mystery of your core muscles.

Checking out your core muscles

To identify the core muscles shown in Figure 2-1, please read the following to gain a better understanding of what muscles you'll be using when you're working on getting that six pack.

The core is so much more than the rectus abdominus and the erector spinea — I mean, the abs and back. The core also includes all the muscles that lie deep within the midsection or torso, from the hips (pelvis) all the way up to and including the neck and shoulders. These muscles lying deep within the core include:

- **Multifidus:** The deep spinal muscles that run segmentally from the neck to the sacrum or the center bone in the chest.

- **External obliques:** The side waist muscles or abdominal muscles that attach at the lower ribs, pelvis, and abdominal fascia.

- **Internal obliques:** The internal waist muscles or abdominal muscles that attach at the lower ribs, rectus sheath, pelvis, and thoracolumbar fascia.

- **Transversus abdominis:** The abdominal muscles that attach at the lower ribs, pelvis, thoracolumbar fascia, and rectus sheath.

   The external obliques, internal obliques, and transverses abdominus all work together as abdominal muscles that stabilize the lumbar spine.

- **Rectus abdominis:** The one you've heard of the most and referred to as "abs" is the primary abdominal muscle that attaches to the lower sternum and the front of the pubic bone. It stretched the entire length of the torso and most people think there are two sets of upper and lower abs but there really is just one — and it can be exercised with only one exercise.

- **Erector spinae:** Better known as the spine — these muscles attach at the base of the skull.

- **Quadratus lumborum:** This muscle actually stabilizes the lumbar spine and helps it "flex" in all directions.

- **Latissimus dorsi:** My favorite! Referred to as the lats — this muscle is the largest spinal stabilizer and helps perform all the pulling motions through the arms. When you work your lats you get a nice "v" shape in your upper back, which makes you look like you have a smaller waist! That's why it's my fave!

- **Thoracolumbar fascia:** Something like a net, this connects and holds the lats, glutes (butt), internal obliques, and transverse abdominis, and supports the spine. It's very important to your body but not as recognized as the glutes!

✔ **Abdominal fascia:** Like a network of wires, these muscles connect the obliques and rectus abdominis to the pecs or pectoralis major.

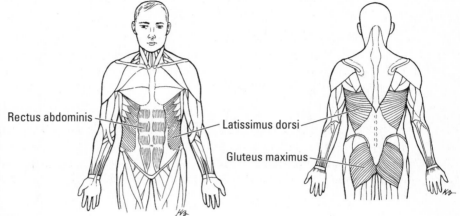

Rectus abdominis

Latissimus dorsi

Gluteus maximus

Figure 2-1: Muscles used for assisting core training.

What is core stabilization and where can I get some?

Core stabilization is the expression used for how the muscles in your trunk keep your spine and your body stable. When all the muscles in your core work together, you'll see the following results:

✔ Better posture

✔ More powerful and efficient movements

✔ A more balanced body

✔ Fewer injuries

✔ Tighter internal and external muscles

✔ Better control over your extremities (arms and legs)

My favorite core stabilizers

I picked three of my favorite core stabilizing muscles to give you an example of what they are and how they assist your core. There are many more but these are the ones I like to exercise the most because they make a big difference in how my core looks and feels — strong!

Rectus abdominus

The rectus abdominus is actually a long, flat muscle that extends across the entire length of the front of the abdomen. It is separated in the middle by the linea alba, which is translated as "white line."

Most commonly referred to as "abs," the rectus abdominus is the muscle responsible for flexing the lumbar spine when doing a sit-up. Terms such as *six-pack* and *washboard abs* apply to the rectus abdominus muscle . . . and, yes, you need to be familiar with this muscle if you're going to be doing core exercises because you'll be calling upon the rectus abdominus a lot!

Latissimus dorsi

Want a tiny waist? Work your latissimus dorsi, better known as "lats." The latissimus dorsi is the back area that looks bumpy when women wear their bras too tight. It runs from your armpit to your butt and also incorporates your midback for doing exercises targeted at the lats. This region is one of my favorites to work out because it makes my waist look so much smaller!

Gluteus maximus

The gluteus maximus, better known as glutes, is one of the largest and strongest muscles in the body. It starts at the pelvic bone and attaches to the rear side of the femur. The glutes are made up of three muscles, actually: the maximus, the medius, and the minimus. The medius and the minimus both lie directly underneath the maximus. (All sounds so Latin, doesn't it?) And the medius and the minimus both start at the same point as the maximus but (no pun intended!) attach to the side of the femur instead of the rear of the femur.

Definitely the powerhouse of the body, the butt, the glutes, the booty — whatever you want to call it — is a strong muscle to help with core stabilization.

Technically speaking . . . opposites attract!

If you've ever wondered what makes your muscles move and the doctor inside you is dying to know how the muscles technically work, here's a breakdown on the way your body makes the majority of its movements:

A primary muscle or the agonist, is assisted by one or more secondary muscles or the synergists; together they stretch the opposing muscle which is the antagonist.

As an example of this, when you bend your knee, the muscles on the back of your leg, including your hamstring (which would be the agonist) and your gastrocnemius (your calf, which would be the synergist) contract, and in turn stretches the quadriceps (the antagonist).

Another example would be during a biceps curl, the biceps is the agonist and the triceps is the antagonist . . . sounds a lot like my ex-husband!

Uncovering Key Core Principles

What makes a healthy core? For that matter, what makes a healthy body? Well, you can take a few steps to enhance your health and your core training. I've listed a few principles that can keep your new core program running solidly and smoothly:

- ✔ **Release it and let it go.** Don't hold muscle tension in your body! If your muscles are constantly in a state of contraction, you can never increase in strength and flexibility. Try to exercise in a state of relaxation, to see the full benefits of strengthening your core. If you hold tension in your glutes, be sure to release it before you start each repetition so that you will see and feel the changes in your body faster.

- ✔ **Be aware of body awareness.** Pay attention to what is happening in your body and with your muscles as you are exercising. Be mindful of your movements and think about the muscle you are working. It helps to visualize each body part as you contract it and focus all your energy on that area. Try it; it really does make a difference.

- ✔ **Choose the best lifestyle possible.** Life is all about making choices, isn't it? So why not make the best choices for you? Eating right and exercising regularly are what I like to call "lifetime commitments to fitness." And that's what I want for you . . . to make a lifetime commitment to fitness! Nobody's perfect, so don't be too hard on yourself. But do try to stay motivated. Before you know it, you'll be motivating others.

- ✔ **Warm up properly.** When the muscles and connective tissues around a muscle are warm, they work better. Increasing your internal temperature and getting your heart rate up are imperative before exercising. You can avoid injury and set yourself up for the best workout ever with a good warm-up.

Benefits of having less belly fat

Reducing belly fat or abdominal fat through core training doesn't just help your figure. It also reduces your risk of disease — and that's good news! If you're a man with a waist larger than 40 inches, it's time to get up and get moving. If you're a woman with a waist size greater than 35 inches, you need to do the same. The inherent risks of being overweight, especially in the belly area, are associated with type 2 diabetes, high blood pressure, and high cholesterol, which puts you at risk for heart disease. The strange thing is, it doesn't happen all at once. If you gain only 2 pounds a year, by the end of ten years, you will be 20 pounds heavier! And that kind of weight gain is detrimental to your health and to your body.

Breathing with Core Muscles for Better Results

One of the most important benefits of exercise is its ability to promote relaxation not only of your body, but of your mind and spirit as well. You would expect that exercise and the release of endorphins can help individual muscles release tension and relax, but the deep, regular breathing that is so important to effective exercise can also oxygenate your blood and produce a reduction in overall stress and anxiety.

Believe it or not, humans breathe in and out more than 20,000 times a day, and yet most people do it incorrectly. I hear you asking right now, how is it possible to breathe wrong? Air goes in, air goes out. Pretty simple, right? Well, not so quick. Because of poor posture or lack of body awareness you end up using the wrong muscles to breathe, which results in shallow, ineffective breathing, and robs you of the full benefits of your breath. In this section, I explain to you not only what muscles you need to use to breathe most effectively, but I also give a foolproof method for taking good core breaths.

The lung itself has no muscles, so it's totally dependent on the muscles around it to create the respiratory process of inhaling and exhaling. This respiratory process can happen in one of two ways:

- ✔ By using the muscles that lift and lower the ribcage — the shoulders and chest
- ✔ By using the muscles of the diaphragm

Unfortunately, most people use the muscles of their shoulders and chest to inhale and exhale. Although these muscles are large and powerful, breathing is not really what they were designed for. Instead, the primary location of the movement of respiration should be the diaphragm, which only has one function: breathing (see Chapter 12).

A full, deep breath can enhance your exercise experience by helping your body to relax and by oxygenating your muscles to increase their performance. Just remember, to get all these wonderful benefits, you need to breathe the way your body was designed — from your core.

To take a full, deep breath from you core, follow these steps:

1. **Inhale through your nose** so that your nose can filter and warm the air before using it.

2. **Exhale through your mouth,** consciously using your deep abdominal muscles and diaphragm to push the air out.

Of course, even if you follow the right steps to a proper core breath, you can further enhance your breathing by maintaining good posture. A rounded back, dropped shoulders, and a forward head can reduce the ability of the diaphragm to contract and the ribs to expand to their full potential. So, sit up or stand up tall with your shoulders back and eyes gazing straight forward to help with good posture and aid in taking the perfect breath.

Testing Your Core Strength

The very best motivation to stick with an exercise program is to see results, which is why I've developed a core self-test. This test simply and easily accomplishes two important goals:

- ✔ To give you a good indication of where you're weak and where your imbalances might be so you know where to focus your strengthening program
- ✔ To mentally track and record your increases in strength over time so you can see how far you've come.

Developing core strength will not happen overnight. Set realistic goals and start with easy exercises before moving on to the more advanced ones. Because no two people are alike some people may see results more quickly and dramatically than others, but as long as you're seeing improvement and enjoying yourself you'll have a much better chance of making exercise a life-long program, which is what it's all about.

In the following sections, I not only list what you need to have to get started with core testing, but I take you through each exercise so that you can plainly see which areas of your body need the most attention.

Getting what you need to test your core

When you first do this self-test it will probably take you about 15 minutes or so to complete. Eventually, after you've begun core training and come back to it, you will be more familiar with the exercises and using proper form, so it'll take you less time.

To get started I suggest that you use the following:

- ✔ Comfortable, breathable, and loose fitting clothes.
- ✔ An exercise mat or carpeted floor. You will need a space large enough to lie down comfortably.

✔ Firm chair or exercise bench.

✔ Sturdy pair of tennis shoes.

✔ A five- to ten-pound pair of dumbbells.

You'll have better results if you're warm before you attempt the test exercises later in this section. Head to Chapter 4 for a few examples of warming up.

Using your results to design a program

I know that taking tests is nobody's favorite thing to do, but you can make this one fun because you know it will result in a stronger core. Performing exercises that involve more than one muscle group at a time makes it difficult to determine which muscle is tight or is causing the weakness in your body. My test exercises isolate individual muscles to give you the most useful information possible to design your own customized core-strengthening program.

After you've done the self-test, you will know exactly what muscles need the most attention. Then simply go to the chapter containing specific core exercises for that area and choose the one that feels most comfortable for your body.

Also, you may notice that most of the core test exercises use both the right and left side of your body. It's not uncommon to have one side of your body that's stronger than the other but it's important to try to get both sides equal in core stabilization and to create good symmetry and balance in the body.

T-raises: Testing your upper back and chest

It is so important to test your strength in your upper back and chest to see if you have what it takes to start core training. Don't forget to pull in your abdominal muscles before trying this one.

This test exercise requires you to pull your weights straight up directly through the centerline or midsection of your body. It will test the strength in your chest, arms, shoulders, and upper back as well.

To do this test exercise, follow these steps:

1. **Standing tall and holding your weights down at your sides, slowly raise your weights until they're straight out in front of you at chest level (as shown in Figure 2-2a).**

2. **Then like an airplane or a "T," move your arms out to either side of your body (see Figure 2-2b).**

3. **Return to starting position by bringing your arms back into the centerline of your chest using a "T" shape, before lowering your weights back down to your sides.**

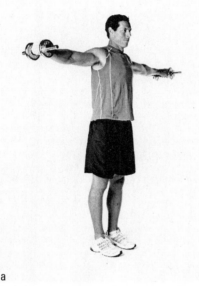 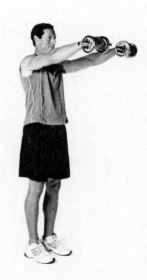

Figure 2-2:
T-raises to
test chest
and upper
back core
strength.

a   b

When you perform this test exercise:

- ✔ Keep your back straight during this exercise.

- ✔ Avoid letting your arms move above your shoulders with the weights.

- ✔ Pull in your abs or pretend you're tightening your belt during this test exercise.

Seated core rotation: Testing the trunk or midsection

Core stabilization describes how the muscles of your trunk help keep your body and spine stable. Core stabilization helps you stay balanced when you move. It's difficult to isolate the muscles of your trunk because many muscles are involved in the complex movement of your spine. Therefore the next test exercise will measure the range of motion you have in your trunk as a whole.

The biggest benefit to having strong lower back muscles is being less prone to injury. Plus, strong abdominal muscles mean stronger back muscles because these muscle groups work together to form the core of the body.

The seated core rotation actually increases the rotational movement in your spine, which in turn helps you acquire strength and flexibility in your trunk by stretching out your lower back muscles.

To do this test core exercise, follow these steps:

1. **Sit up tall on a sturdy chair with your feet flat on the floor and close together, knees at a right angle.**
2. **Anchor your right hand on the side of the chair as you place your left hand on the outside of your right thigh (see Figure 2-3a).**
3. **Inhale and as you exhale, twist your torso to the right, and look back over your shoulder (see Figure 2-3b).**
4. **Hold the exercise for about ten seconds.**

   Try to make a mental note of a stationary object you see that's about at eye level.
5. **Release and come back to center.**
6. **Inhale again, and as you exhale repeat on the opposite side.**

   Find the same object you were looking at, but this time try to find another object that's past it.

While doing the seated core rotation, remember to:

- ✔ Keep your feet flat on the floor.
- ✔ Keep your knees and feet together and facing the front.
- ✔ Avoid forcing the stretch or pulling too hard on the back of the chair.
- ✔ Find an object that's at eye level — don't look down.

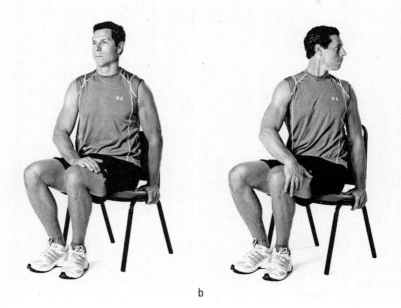

Figure 2-3:
Seated core
rotation.

a   b

Back and butt extensions:
Testing the buttocks

The largest muscle of the body that helps move you and helps with core stabilization are the muscles in your buttocks — now see, you weren't just imagining that your behind was the biggest thing on your body! Your buttock muscles combined with the back muscles, pelvis, and hips on the other side of your body are the powerhouse or core stabilizers.

Core stabilization strengthens the muscles of the buttocks and teaches you to use the inner muscles before you start to move with the outer muscles. When doing butt exercises, the focus becomes on smooth coordinated movement along with the muscles of your back.

This back and butt test exercise seems simple yet it is a powerful and effective back and butt strengthener. It targets the lower back and your butt when you squeeze it tight to keep your core lifted off the floor.

To do this test exercise, follow these steps:

1. **Using a mat or towel, lie on your stomach placing your arms at your sides with palms facing up (see Figure 2-4a).**

2. **Pulling in or contracting your abdominal muscles, lift your chest a few inches off the floor keeping your gaze straight ahead at all times (see Figure 2-4b).**

3. **Hold for a few seconds before lowering your chest back toward the ground.**

   Repeat this test a few times.

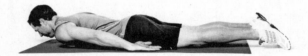

a

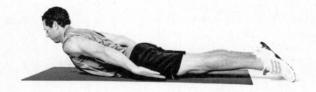

Figure 2-4:
Core test
for buttocks
and back.

b

While doing back and butt extensions, keep these tips in mind:

✔ Tighten your butt or glutes to protect your lower back as you lift your chest off the floor.

✔ Tighten your abdominals throughout this move.

✔ Lift only to the point that you're not straining your back — don't lift too high off the floor.

Chapter 3

Getting Started: Your Core Guidelines

In This Chapter

▶ Getting the most out of your core-strengthening program

▶ Finding out what makes up a healthy core

▶ Using proper exercise technique to acquire core strength

▶ Determining your fitness level with some basic testing

Yep — sit-ups suck! And so does most core work. But if you have a weak core, everything else in your body will suffer. On the other hand, strengthening your core helps your body bridge the gap between the upper and lower body by enhancing your movements and creating good form. Your posture, your spine, and your backbone all line up better with core training and help all of your sports and functional movements become more efficient. And along with core strength comes an improvement in all sports and functional movements you use throughout the day. In this chapter, I lay out core guidelines for you to follow as you work your way through this book.

Finding Your Fitness Level

You need to know whether you can even begin core training, let alone where you can begin. Determining where you need to be with this program (or whether you're fit enough to begin it in the first place) is important. You want to minimize your risk of injury by starting with the proper amount of exercise. For example, if you work out at a moderate level, you may be able to do two sets of abdominal crunches instead of just one, as I prescribe for beginners in this book.

The following sections give you some questions to ask yourself to determine whether you're ready to start and, if so, how much you should be doing.

Determining whether you're ready to begin

Some of you may work out daily, and some of you may not work out at all. However, because I don't know you personally or know where you are physically in your exercise regime, you need to answer a few questions before you can begin core training.

So wherever you are on your path to fitness, take a moment to ask yourself the following questions:

- ✔ Do you breathe heavily when walking up stairs?
- ✔ Do you experience chest pains before, during, or after exercising?
- ✔ Do you have any injuries that would prevent you from exercising proper form when beginning a new workout?
- ✔ Do you take prescription medication for heart disease or high blood pressure?
- ✔ Do you get dizzy when exercising?

If you answered *yes* to any of the above questions, ask your doctor before beginning any exercise. As the saying goes, "An ounce of prevention is worth a pound of cure." I call this preventive medicine, so consult your doctor before you get started, just to be safe!

Figuring out where to start

Everyone wants to be advanced and jump right in to every exercise with the ability to rip off 30 reps without any trouble. But the reality is, not quite everyone falls into that category. If you know (or your doctor has told you) you're healthy enough to begin core training, find out whether you're a beginner, intermediate, or advanced exerciser. I've included some questions to help you determine where you fall. You may be wondering why I left out "intermediate" . . . well, I didn't. If you fall somewhere between the guidelines for beginner and advanced, consider yourself intermediate.

Ask yourself the following questions to find out where your fitness level falls:

- ✔ How often do you work out? To keep your body from detraining or breaking down precious muscle, you want to exercise at least three times a week consistently. Using that as your gauge, determine where you are on your path to fitness and go from there.

  - **Beginner:** If you paused a moment to think about it, I'm going to take a chance here and put you in the beginner category.

- **Intermediate/advanced:** If your answer is that you exercise three to five times per week, I will be putting you in the intermediate to advanced category. You should also have be working out consistently for 6 to 12 months to make this more advanced category and have seen some significant changes in your body along with a greater endurance level.

✔ **How much cardio do you get?** Aerobic exercise is really important for good circulation and to help maintain a healthy heart. Cardio activity provides oxygen to your blood, and blood pumping through your veins keeps everything running smoothly — and helps you sleep better, too!

- **Beginner:** If you're doing only 60 to 90 minutes of cardio a week, you have room for improvement and I would place you in the beginner category.

- **Intermediate/advanced:** If you're walking regularly for 30 minutes daily, that's excellent! In fact, walking is my favorite form of aerobic exercise. I prescribe walking to all age groups and demographics, no matter what stage of life they're in.

How often do you engage in strength or resistance training?

- **Beginner:** If you haven't used weights, you are definitely a beginner and need to start (check out the sidebar "Osteoporosis," later in this chapter). Any form of strength training enhances your health, speeds up weight loss, and builds a healthier body. Using your own body weight as resistance, such as performing push-ups or dips, is fantastic, too. You need a certain amount of strength in your back and abdominals to begin, so start slowly with core training and give yourself time to build up strength as you progress through the exercises in this book.

- **Intermediate/advanced:** A good rule of thumb is, if you've been regularly doing strength training for at least three months, you're good to go with core training and are in the intermediate to advanced category.

✔ **How often do you stretch?** Not stretching and just doing strength-training exercises and cardio creates an imbalance in your body. To prevent injuries and learn how to maintain balance, you have to do some stretching.

- **Beginner:** If you're new to stretching and your range of motion is very limited, put yourself in the beginner category and build your flexibility slowly by holding the stretches in this book only until you feel comfortable.

- **Intermediate/advanced:** If you regularly take yoga or Pilates classes are flexible enough to touch your toes or place the palms of your hands on the floor, your are definitely in the intermediate/ advanced category.

Picking Up Pointers for Your Level of Fitness

If you know your level of fitness (if not, read through the section "Finding Your Fitness Level," earlier in this chapter, to find out), check out the following information so you know how often and how hard you should be working.

Core training two times per week is best for all levels, along with some form of cardio training three times a week. That regimen makes up a really well-rounded workout and also makes for a well-rounded derriere!

Beginners

If you decide you're at the beginner level for core strengthening, start by doing ten repetitions. Also start by doing only one set; you can add a set when you feel that you've fully mastered using the proper form while performing the core exercises. Listen to your body and move forward when you feel it's time to increase your level of resistance.

Intermediate

If you've decided that you're ready to work at the intermediate level, doing 15 repetitions is best for you. Start by doing only one set of core exercises; if you feel that you're using proper form and are ready to take on another set, go for it. If that feels like too much for your body, complete two weeks of training before you add another set of 15 repetitions to each exercise.

Advanced

If you're exercising at an advanced level, start with 20 repetitions. You can also start by doing two sets instead of just one; you're starting off in great shape and looking to enhance what you already have.

You'll also want to do the advanced version of each core exercise, to challenge yourself and see results faster.

Osteoporosis

Osteoporosis is a common condition that can occur when the bone tissue in our bodies breaks down faster than our bodies can build it. As a result, the bones become thin and brittle. Osteoporosis strikes 80 percent of women and 20 percent of men in a population of 10 million. And this condition is growing fast, with 34 million Americans expected to be at risk of osteoporosis as a result of low bone mass.

Women have less bone mass than men, mainly because of hormones, and they experience an accelerated loss when they go through menopause.

To slow the process, you can do a few things:

✔ Perform weight-bearing exercises regularly.

✔ Make sure you're getting the right amount of calcium and vitamin D in your diet.

✔ Don't smoke!

✔ Don't drink too much alcohol. The American Heart Association recommends one 8-ounce glass of red wine daily to keep your heart healthy.

Your doctor can prescribe medicine that you can take to increase bone mass, especially after menopause. To find out if you need to be taking any kind of medication for bone loss, get a bone density test from your doctor.

Getting Your Muscles to Chill Out

Often when you exercise, you focus on how *much* you can do, but you really should focus on how *safely* you exercise. Tensing up your muscles when exercising can lead to an injury and place undue strain on all the surrounding muscles and other body parts. So keeping your muscles tension-free helps to prevent injury, which at the same time helps you reach your ultimate fitness goals. To keep the tension out of your muscles while exercising, keep these important safety precautions in mind:

✔ **Take a break as soon as you recognize that you're losing your form.** When you feel you're losing your form while you're doing a particular exercise, your body is giving you a signal that it's time to stop. You have to listen to your body and read your body's signals so that you know when your body is telling you that it has had enough.

✔ **Keep your muscles relaxed.** Instead of tensing your muscles, like hunching up your shoulders when you're exercising, use the strength of your muscles to propel or push you through each movement without tensing them up.

Headache relief from strained and sore muscles

Statistics show that over 90 percent of people have a headache at some time in their life, which, amazingly, means that a lucky 10 percent of people never have a headache (sounds weird to me). But a headache can happen at any time, anywhere, and can definitely ruin your day. And even though headaches are common, most people don't have any idea where a headache comes from.

Tension headaches are by far the most common form of headaches, and can be due to stress, which causes you to clench or strain the muscles of your face, neck, jaw, and/or shoulders. When these muscles are tight they can compress the nerves that lead to your scalp, causing a tight, squeezing sensation in your head. Fatigue, lack of sleep, or even sleep disorders can also result in this type of headache.

Posture also plays a key role in many tension headaches. Many of the positions we habitually put ourselves in tighten neck and back muscles. Try to avoid constantly tilting your head to one side (a problem for frequent phone users). Be aware of your posture as you sit at your desk, drive your car, stand in line at the grocery store, or carry a bag or purse.

Migraines are generally less common headaches but more severe. Although stress can be a major trigger for migraine headache, migraines and cluster headaches are regarded as primarily vascular in nature, and not necessarily the result of muscle tightness. What triggers a migraine headache in one person may have no effect in someone else, including hormone fluctuations, smoking, chocolate, and even the weather.

When it comes to relieving the pain of occasional tension headaches, thousands of people turn to over-the-counter drugs such as aspirin, acetaminophen, or ibuprofen, which can be very effective. In addition, some proven-effective natural remedies include

- Ice packs
- A warm shower or bath
- Massaging the neck and shoulders
- Aerobic exercise (to promote the release of endorphins and relax tight muscles)
- Eating regularly
- Sex
- A glass of wine

Treatment for recurrent tension headaches, however, is another story. A frequently throbbing head is your body's way of telling you that something significant is out of balance in your life. Stress is an unavoidable part of modern life, but by far the best course of action to combat stress-related tension headaches is prevention. Although such natural remedies as a visit to a chiropractor, acupressure, acupuncture, and even hypnosis can help with recurring tension headaches, several well-regarded studies have concluded that stress management skills and relaxation training can reduce chronic headache for 50 to 70 percent of patients. Techniques such as deep breathing, meditation, and, most important of all, exercise and deep stretching can trigger the relaxation response, which can lower blood pressure, reduce pulse rates, and release muscle tension. Regular exercise and stretching keeps you calm and flexible; and it can help reduce headache frequency and intensity.

✔ **Remember to breathe.** Focus on your breathing (read the section later on in this chapter, "Breathing Properly for Better Results") using slow and steady breaths. The worst thing you can do is to hold your breath, which some people tend to do when they exercise. Using your breath will help keep you focused on your body and the movements you are doing with your body.

✔ **Warm up and cool down properly.** As I mention throughout this book (see Chapter 4), warming up for 5 to 10 minutes before working out prepares your body for exercise by getting your blood circulating and increasing your core temperature slowly. The same goes for cooling down properly, which reduces your risk of injury and helps the blood return to your heart.

Benefits of Stretching Your Core (or Anything, for That Matter)

Have you ever seen anyone in great shape who slouches when sitting? Obviously, this person toned and tightened his or her body but forgotten to lengthen it. Stretching adds great form and definition to a body that's already well toned. And you really can't get that look with short, round, compact muscles. So read on to find the many other benefits of stretching out the new six-pack (or, at least, flat tummy) you'll get after reading this book.

Beats stress

Stretching beats stress. Yay! Now that's a reason to cheer or stretch! Of course, some stress can be good and can help keep you motivated so you can take action and achieve great things. But too much stress can threaten your health and well-being. We all have to learn ways of coping with stress, and stretching can be therapeutic for many people. Stretching can help individual muscles release and relax, but the deep, regular breathing that is so important to effective stretching can also oxygenate your blood and reduce overall stress and anxiety. What's more, the slow, meticulous movements in a good flexibility program can provide a meditative effect. So increase your focus and your range of motion with a little stretching.

Gives you great posture

Not only can sound, erect posture make you look taller and thinner, but it is also essential to allow your body to perform the way it was meant to. What's more, good posture aids dramatically in facilitating free and effective breathing. The main enemy of good posture is tight muscles! Stretching can help you correct muscular imbalances that lead to incorrect skeletal alignment. One cause of this kind of imbalance is using one side of your body more than the other — like when you carry your toddler on the same side, or always carry your briefcase in the same hand, or perhaps even wearing your shoulder bag on the same shoulder. Such chronic imbalances can rob you of energy and efficiency from movement or even result in back pain. Stretching regularly can help balance out these bad habits, so be sure to stand up straight and stretch!

Increases your range of motion

Just as stretching can help dramatically increase the range of motion in your joints, it can also help in your everyday life by making it possible for you to reach higher or lower, bend farther, and reduce nagging aches and pains from tight, tense muscles. A lack of flexibility can make small everyday movements annoying and even painful. Stretching is the perfect means of improving your functional flexibility, and it helps the day go smoother.

Prevents injuries

Stretching has been proven to reduce muscle strain or joint strain, in the case of accidental overuse of muscles or joints from sports. In short, although nothing can prevent an injury 100 percent, numerous studies show that, with stretching exercises, you can increase flexibility and decrease your risk of injury. In the end, stretching can be a very low-cost, long-term insurance policy for your body — and well worth the few minutes a day it takes to do it!

Stretching Do's and Don'ts

Trainers sometimes have quite different opinions on when to stretch (before or after a workout) and sometimes even on the benefits of stretching. So to avoid any misunderstanding on where I stand on stretching and just how important it is (did I mention I wrote *Stretching For Dummies*?), I put together a list of stretching do's and don'ts to explain it all. The following guidelines help you get started so you can begin stretching out your core after you take a look at my simple rules!

Do stretch after your workout

The time to stretch is when your muscles are warm! A lot of trainers will tell you to stretch either first thing in the morning, or at the end of the day, or both. And although some research supports this recommendation, I always recommend stretching after the body is warmed up. "Always better to error on the side of caution" is another one of my favorite sayings. Be safe and increase your flexibility by ending every workout with a few nice stretches, like the ones you find in this chapter.

Do stretch a little bit every other day

If you're looking to increase your present level of flexibility (and who isn't?), I recommend that you engage in a focused flexibility program every other day. To increase flexibility in a muscle, the general rule is to stretch that muscle at least once a day, but most of us don't have the luxury of that much time. I'm confident that you can maintain a great range of motion by stretching every other day. Of course, that means after your body is warmed up from gardening, walking up a hill, taking a hike, or finishing up a great swim session.

Do hold each stretch

Many studies have demonstrated that the optimum effectiveness of a stretching exercise is reached only after holding that stretch for approximately 30 seconds. If you stretch any less, you don't really give your body time to adapt properly to the stretch. (Stretching more hasn't been proven to provide any additional benefits, either.) So if you stick to the 30-second rule — or about five or six good, deep breaths — you'll be right where you need to be and will feel a difference in your flexibility in no time.

Don't stretch to the point of pain

"No pain, no gain" is definitely not the saying for anyone who's stretching, and neither is "Go for the burn." In fact, pain is the most precise indicator of a stretch that has gone too far, in either intensity or duration. If you're stretching to the point at which your muscle is quivering or you actually find that you are becoming less flexible, back off. A stretch should feel no more than slightly uncomfortable. When you reach the point of resistance in your muscle, stay there and hold the stretch at that point. You'll find that you can comfortably move past that point in a few days. However, if you force the issue, it'll only set you back further than you were when you started.

Do start at the top of the body and work your way down

Progressing through a series of body parts that starts at the top of your head and ends at the tip of your toes helps the muscles warm up and increases flexibility in the best way possible.

The following sequence shows you which body part is best to start with and which one to end with. This guide is only a small one, but I think it will help you to stretch safely, starting with the smallest muscle groups and then working up to the largest muscle groups in your body:

- Neck
- Forearm and wrists
- Triceps
- Chest
- Back
- Sides (obliques)
- Buttocks (gluteals)
- Groin
- Thighs
- Calves
- Shins
- Hamstrings

Chapter 4

Things to Consider Before Taking the Core Challenge

So you want to get rid of that "muffin top," and that's why you're reading this book, right? I remember when I first heard that expression — muffin top — you know, the fat that spills over the top of your buttoned jeans. Yikes! And wouldn't life be great if only you could get rid of it? Well, you've come to the right place! This book will not only help you feel better, but will also help you become a sleeker version of your former self (or at least help you button your jeans).

Of course, you'll want to know a few points before you get started, the most important being that you should get your doctor's approval before starting any new workout program. And when you have the go-ahead, you can check out this chapter to find out how to warm up your core temperature first for a better, safer workout. Plus, you can discover many ways to add weights to your core workout, and even try out a core class.

Tuning In to Toning-Up Basics

Core training may be new to you, or you may be ready to up your core workout with some new, more intense moves. Regardless of where you're starting, you need to be sure that you understand some of the basics of core training before you begin. The following sections give you all the info you need to grasp the core basics, including everything from warming up and building a proper workout to practicing core safety.

Turning up the heat of your core

Like most people, you're probably rushed and don't feel you have the time to warm up, so you just dive right into working out, right? Or you've been given mixed advice on whether to warm up before a workout. Well, never fear, because I'm here to tell you that you must *always* warm up before exercising. The following list explains the benefits of a proper warm-up:

- **Getting some internal heat going:** To improve exercise performance and get your blood flowing (which pumps more oxygen to your muscles for a high-energy workout), you have to do five to ten minutes of light aerobic activity. Warming up your muscles properly with simple movements like marching or jogging in place helps prevent the possibility of injury due to cold muscles because warmer muscles work more efficiently than cold ones.

- **Improving your concentration:** Don't rush the warm-up. Taking your time when you're warming up helps your mind to focus and signals the body that it's time to get going. Warming up slowly improves your concentration and increases brain wave activity, to help make the transition to a high-energy workout safer and easier. So no matter how rushed for time you are or how much you feel you can skip the warm-up, don't. You'll have a much better workout if you do.

Knowing your limits

Core training can be very intense, so start slowly. Pushing past your limit can cause injury or, at the very least, pain. In particular, two factors can lead to headaches and sore muscles:

- **Jumping right into a new workout:** Just because you run every day doesn't mean that you can do 50 crunches and not feel a thing. The body needs time to learn new movements, and working different muscle groups challenges you in a whole new way. So avoid the tendency to do too much right from the start. Work up slowly, to avoid injury and get the best results.

- **Not staying well hydrated:** When you're ready to work up a good sweat, you'll need to have a bottle of water handy so you can drink frequently, to replace what you lose during the sweating process.

In addition to taking your time and staying well hydrated, you need to understand when you're reaching your limit so you can back off. The following list gives you an idea of when your body is telling you to slow down:

✔ You feel dizzy or lose your balance

✔ You can't carry on a conversation or sing Happy Birthday!

✔ You feel a sharp pain anywhere in your body

Setting aside enough time for working out

When it comes to working out, people often cite time as the primary reason they can't fit in a workout. But if you work efficiently and follow the ideas for putting together a proper workout, you can find plenty of spots to fit it in during the day. For every workout, be sure to

✔ **Include a warm-up before *every* workout that consists of five to ten minutes** of movement, to increase your core temperature and to prepare your body for the exercises that are about to come.

✔ **For your actual workout, strive for at least 30 minutes** three times a week to start your new core program. Because you use your deeper abdominal muscles (which you probably haven't used before) when you do core training, your body will feel the difference right away and be a bit sore from your ribs to your hips. Resting for 48 hours between workouts gives your body a chance to replenish and recharge. If you still feel some soreness after you rest for 48 hours in between your workouts, I recommend working a different part of your body or a different muscle group entirely, to prevent any additional damage to the area. Make sure you drink a lot of water, to aid in tissue repair, and try gentle stretching (Check out *Stretching For Dummies* [Wiley], by yours truly!) until you feel ready to start again.

✔ **Cool down properly** after working out, by stretching your muscles to relieve any tightness you may have and to reduce your risk of injury. A five-minute cooldown will help the blood flow back to your brain and reduce your risk of dizziness. It also gives the body a chance to slow down your rate of breathing and sends a signal to your body that you are done with exercising so you can begin breathing normally.

As you become more proficient with your core exercises, you can increase your workouts to 60 minutes three to four days a week by adding some form of cardio for 30 to 40 minutes. Adding cardio, provides you with faster results by helping you burn more calories to get rid of that "muffin top" and boosting your metabolism.

Keeping core safety in mind

For the safest and most effective workout, follow these simple and easy tips:

- ✔ **Use a smooth and steady motion for each exercise.** When you're doing any form of resistance training for core strengthening, maintaining good posture and control is important. Whether you're lifting weights or doing crunches, controlling the movement — and not letting the movement control you — is the key. If you start to lose your form, you're doing your body a disservice and you may injure yourself.

- ✔ **Breathe freely while exercising.** Never hold your breath while working out. Breathing freely helps you gain better control of your movements.

- ✔ **Remember to stay within your own limits.** Never try an exercise that may risk you hurting yourself or pulling a muscle.

- ✔ **If you feel any kind of pain — especially in your joints — never continue the exercise.** Remember that a sharp pain is different from the slight pain or fatigue that you feel in your muscles when you're "going for the burn." Some exercises in this book may just not feel right for your particular body, so move on to find the ones that do.

- ✔ **Perform the exercises in this book only in the ways in which they're demonstrated.** Adding your own little twist to proven and effective exercises can cause injury. Stick within the guidelines for each exercise, and you'll be fit to the core in no time!

- ✔ **Stay within your training range.** When you begin working out after taking a long time off, going a little nutty and doing too much is easy to do. When you're just beginning, staying within your own level of comfort and not lifting too heavy a load keeps you from getting an injury and hindering your progress. If you're consistent with your exercise program, you'll see results in a few short weeks.

- ✔ **If you feel dizzy or short of breath, stop the exercise.** Because core training uses many lying positions that you will be sitting up from, you can easily become dizzy. If you experience dizziness or shortness of breath, stop immediately and breathe deeply while you rest.

- ✔ **Exercise in an open space.** Never exercise in a confined or limited space. Remember to remove anything with sharp edges from your workout area, to keep yourself from running into anything when you exercise.

- ✔ **Always consult your doctor to make sure that you're in good physical shape before you begin a new exercise program.** In addition, if you have a history of back or neck problems or are pregnant, discuss these issues with your health-care provider to find out if he or she feels that core training is a good choice for you.

In addition, remember to always warm up properly to get your body ready for exercising and to avoid injury. And when you're finished working out, cool down (and stretch) to avoid soreness.

Using a mat

Creating a space to work out, whether it's at home or at the gym, is important for your success. You should include an exercise mat in that space. Taking the pain out of exercising and supporting your body weight with an exercise mat is the best thing you can do for yourself — and your joints.

Doing push-ups on your knees, like I suggest in some chapters, is tough enough without using something to cushion them. So is lying on your back to do bicycles and the other abdominal exercises I prescribe in this book. So grab a yoga mat (ideal), a towel, or similar item, to soften the rough floor and ensure your success as you're doing the exercises in this book.

Using a mirror

Coming from a dance background, I'm used to watching myself in a mirror, to see whether I'm lifting my chest properly, keeping my knees in line, and standing up straight. A mirror is a great tool for making sure that you have the desired neutral alignment of your spine and checking your form throughout many of the exercises contained in this book.

So what kind of mirror works best? For starters, any mirror that's bolted to the wall! You certainly don't want to use a free-standing mirror (like a wardrobe mirror), in case you lose your balance and knock it over. If you have the space in your garage or office, a wall mirror works great for checking your body alignment — and for staying put.

Warming Up Your Core

Both men and women can benefit greatly from warming up first before doing core training, but what are some of the best ways to warm up? You can do one of the following recommended types of warm-ups so you're ready to go.

You're warming up, not working out yet. Start out with a nice gradual pace that you can add on slowly to when you begin your actual workout.

Jogging in place

Ten minutes of jogging in place at a slow pace works great for preparing your body for exercise. Jogging is easy to do, and you don't need much space! Just make sure you don't break into a full-out run; maintain a slower, warm-up pace that helps you break a light sweat by the end of ten minutes.

Marching it out

Marching in place is another easy way to warm up your body. Make sure you lift your knees high enough to get your heart rate up, and pump your arms to incorporate your upper body. Figure 4-1 gives you an idea of what proper marching looks like.

To march, follow these steps:

1. **Standing with your feet together, lift your knees high above your hips.**

2. **Swing your arms up and back, making sure your hands are above your heart.**

3. **Step down, using a flat foot each time, until you work up a light sweat.**

Figure 4-1:
Marching
it out — a
good way
to warm up
from head
to toe.

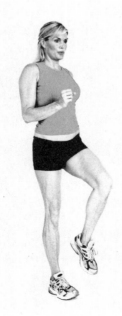

a

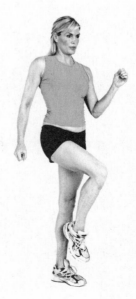

b

Marching in place for five minutes and then walking it out for five minutes back and forth across the room is also a good combination for getting ready to work out.

Jumping rope

My favorite method for warming up the body is jumping rope (see Figure 4-2). You can also pretend you're using a jump rope, which is just as effective for getting in a quick warm-up.

When you jump rope, follow these steps:

1. **Keeping your elbows at your waist, rotate your wrists as you hold the rope in your hands.**

2. **Lift your feet off the ground slightly, or only high enough to allow the rope to slide underneath.**

3. **Bend your knees and jump upward, making sure you land on the balls of your feet.**

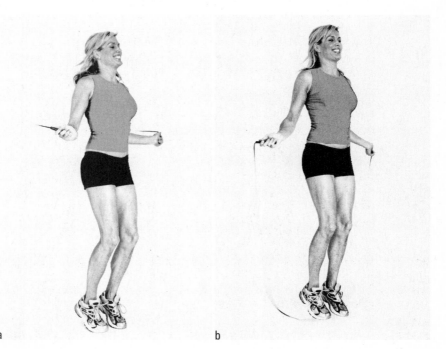

Figure 4-2:
Jumping
rope.

a   b

Always land on the balls of your feet, not your toes, when you're jumping rope.

Holding Your Posture

Having correct posture when performing core exercises is essential. First, correct posture places less stress on your joints; second, it stabilizes your spine, to prevent injury. When you strengthen your core, you'll find that you can stand taller and will have a leaner look overall. This is because certain back muscles are included in the core musculature which can give you a more erect spine and beautiful posture when you strengthen them. The sections that follow introduce you to your neutral spine and explain just how you can find it when you want it.

Achieving a neutral spine

One of the principle factors in core training is using proper back placement, or *neutral spine*. The ultimate goal in trying to achieve a neutral spine is to keep the natural curve of your spine without overcorrecting it, known as the "S" curve.

The "S" shape has three curves, just like neutral spine — one in your neck, one in your upper back, and one in your lower back. In other words, you want to stabilize your back, your hipbones, and your pelvis so they're on the same plane.

If you were standing, your pelvis would drop straight down. The proper way to describe a neutral spine while standing up is a spine that is neither arched nor tilted forward. Just as your car has a neutral position in which it doesn't move forward or backward, the same goes for a neutral spine.

Try standing sideways in front of a mirror to check your posture. Pull your shoulders back and keep your head in line with your spine.

Finding your "hard to find" neutral spine

To try neutral spine and see whether you're maintaining that natural curve in your spine, do the following:

1. **Lie with your back and feet flat on the floor and your knees bent at a 90-degree angle.**

2. **Flatten your lower back by pressing it into the floor.**

   Now you can feel the difference between neutral spine and a flat back.

3. **Arch your back slightly by lifting your hips.**

   Now that you can feel the differences between an arched back and a flat back, you'll find it easier to maintain the natural curve in your spine (or neutral spine).

Knowing how a neutral spine feels

Your core, or midsection (consisting of the abdominal and back muscles), is used in *every* movement you do throughout the day. You've probably heard that a weak back means you have weak abdominals, and that's the best example I can give you to illustrate how much everything in your body is connected and emphasize how important it is to strengthen your core. So what will you feel when you start crunching and bending sideways to improve this area? Check the following sections to see if you're on track and if you're targeting the right muscles that make up your core.

What to feel

If you're lying down on the couch and come to a sitting position, you're using your rectus abdominus. So, for example, when you're doing a crunch, the rectus abdominus helps you move your upper body toward your lower body — and it's better known as the muscle group you need to work out to get a great six-pack! If you find it hard to get up from a lying-down position on the couch, you need to work your core.

You'll get the feeling of wearing a tight girdle when you work the transverse abdominus, or lower abdomen, that supports your spine and internal organs. Together, the upper and lower abdominal areas, or rectus abdominus and transverse abdominus, work to give you a more toned tummy and defined waist so when you lose that layer of fat that covers your midsection, you'll see your new six pack peeking through.

Where to feel it

Your spine, your back, your tummy, your pelvis, your rib cage — you'll start feeling improvements in all these areas when you start core training. Your lower back will feel more steady or stabilized, as if it's working as one unit with the rest of your body. Your neck, or top of the spine, will feel stronger so you can hold your posture erect for longer periods of time. And the spinal vertebrae that run along the entire length of your back will make all your bending movements easier. So prepare to feel more flexible in your entire body and have a more sculpted look throughout the waist area if you're doing core training properly.

How Weights Can Build a Stronger Core

I like to add different kinds of resistance or weights to my core workout, and I think you will, too (see Chapter 10). The trend nowadays is to use free weights or dumbbells and combine exercises, like a squat with an overhead press. When you combine the two movements, you are forced to transition the exercise movement through your core. The core muscles, in turn, help to maintain good posture throughout the exercise. So you can see how one hand helps wash the other — or whatever that saying is!

The following sections provide a few examples of how you can use different forms of weighted resistance to get fit to the core.

When you use hand weights and other accessories, like medicine balls, you need shoes to protect your toes in case you drop a weight on them.

Dumbbells

For men and women who are interested in building muscle mass, heavier dumbbells that allow you to complete only 6 to 12 repetitions comfortably are perfect. However, for core training purposes, and to be able to maintain proper form without straining, use only the amount of weight that feels comfortable to you when performing 10 to 15 repetitions. I suggest 5 to 10 pounds for women and 15 to 25 pounds for men.

Heavy balls (medicine balls)

Heavy balls (medicine balls) are a good accessory to use to increase your resistance and to add some amount of weight to your workout. Heavy balls range in size from a tennis ball to a softball and start out weighing just less than a pound. They continue to increase in size in one-inch increments and are available in different colors to identify their weight and size.

Heavy balls are easier to grip than hand weights because of their round shape, and they provide added resistance to strengthen your core because you can incorporate them more easily into core movements. I like using a five-pound weighted ball or heavy ball that is just a bit smaller than a basketball (see Chapter 9).

Dressing for success: How clothing makes a difference when working out

Although dressing for every kind of sport has become fashionable (tennis wear is suddenly hip), keep some safety considerations in mind before exercising. Because you'll sweat during your workout, breathable cotton is best for keeping you cool and helping you not get too sticky. Bulky clothes and untucked shirts can also bunch up while you're working out, so stick with something form fitting, like what you'd wear to a yoga or Pilates class. This type of clothing allows you to visualize the muscles you're working and focus on your movements better when you can actually see them. You'll also be able to check your posture and study your form better.

No weights

If you're brand new to working out, I recommend not using weights because, although you may have strong muscles on the outside of your body, you probably need to strengthen your inside muscles (or core-stabilizing muscles) first, to develop control over all your movements.

Trying a Core Class

If you're like me, you'll do anything to find a good class. Whether it's kickboxing, spinning, or yoga, I find being in a group class to be very motivating. Okay, so maybe I just get bored when I'm on the elliptical trainer or the treadmill and am forced to watch Montel Williams. Or maybe I just don't have the discipline to go at it alone. But whatever the case may be, group classes are all the rage right now — I suggest trying one as soon as you can!

Check out a few answers to some of the most frequently asked questions about what you should know when you do find a group class for core training:

✔ **Where can I take a class?** Your local YMCA or YWCA is a good place to start looking for a group class. Local gyms and recreational centers also offer classes on a regular basis, depending on the area you live in. You can call your local chamber of commerce to get a list of the fitness facilities in your area that offer classes or search the Internet for a particular location.

✔ **How much does a class cost?** Core classes range in price from $10 to $12 a class, depending on the facility that's offering them. If you're a member of a gym that offers core classes, the cost is most likely included in your monthly payment.

✔ **How long does the class take?** Core-training classes frequently last 30 to 45 minutes these days. Classes begin with a warm-up and end with a cooldown, so your actual workout time is around 25 minutes. Many classes combine other pieces of equipment, like medicine balls and light weights, to help increase core strength.

Some classes incorporate other forms of training; these classes are called *circuit classes.* Circuit classes add accessories (like body bars), dumbbells, and cardio equipment (like jump ropes) to strengthen your body and increase endurance. Circuit classes are also known as boot camp classes because that's just what they are — tough, like a boot camp!

✔ **What kind of teacher should I look for?** Look for a teacher who can teach at all different levels, ranging from beginners to experienced athletes. The teacher should be particularly conscientious of the level of his or her class, to make sure that everyone in the class is using proper form at all times.

Health club providers usually require their instructors to have certifications, including ones from the International Sports Sciences Association, America Council on Exercise, and Aerobics and Fitness Association of America, among others. Resist-A-Ball certifies instructors for core training that consists of different levels and other applications of the exercise ball that they can use with Pilates, yoga, and pregnancy workouts.

✔ **How many times per week should I take a class?** To get the best results, taking a class two or three times per week is best. Combine your core classes with some form of cardio workout, which you can do on your days off from your group class. Walking, jumping rope, spinning, and using the treadmill or an elliptical trainer are all perfect complements to core training.

Finally, consider some friendly group-class reminders to make the transition into an exercise class go a little smoother:

✔ Because some classes require participants to sign up ahead of time, always arrive early to make sure that you have a spot.

✔ Always arrive a few minutes early to class, to give yourself time to get settled in and chose whatever equipment may be needed for the class.

✔ Never enter a class after the warm-up has begun because your body won't be well prepared for that particular workout.

Part II

Core Workouts to Help Sculpt Your Trouble Areas

The 5th Wave   By Rich Tennant

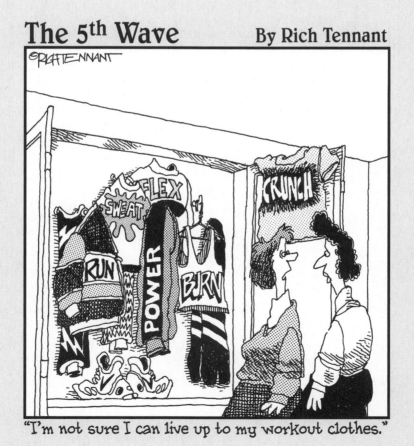

"I'm not sure I can live up to my workout clothes."

In this part . . .

No matter where you're weak, you'll find a core exercise that's right for you in this part. This is where I cover core exercises for every part of your body. I show you beginner exercises for your abs, hips, and back in Chapter 5, before moving on to how to get a six-pack in the aptly titled Chapter 6.

In Chapter 7, I show you core exercises specifically designed for your butt. Finally, in Chapter 8, you'll discover how to put all the core exercises from this part into a killer core routine to strengthen your entire body.

Chapter 5

Getting Started with Beginner Core Exercises

In This Chapter

▶ Getting familiar with doing core exercises

▶ Discovering why using a mat can be good

▶ Creating some simple core strengtheners for your body

▶ Discovering the best core principles for a healthier you

*Y*our core is made up of the muscles of your back, abs, hips, and — well, I like to think of it as anything from the top of your ribcage to the bottom of your hips. Because these core muscles all work together to support your spine, they're the foundation of every movement you do throughout your day, as well as your movements in sports and other activities. So whether you're shooting hoops, gardening, or reaching for something on the top shelf, every movement actually begins with your core.

Because of your body's connection to its core, core training has become very popular and is the foundation of any good fitness program. The following beginner core series includes some basic core exercises, like crunches. Plus, I've added a few back strengtheners to make sure everything is working together, giving you the strongest foundation possible.

Using Everyday Ways to Work Your Core

Challenging your balance works your core — you'll hear these words over and over again when anyone talks about core training. But what does this statement mean to you in real life? Well, challenging your balance simply means you are changing your weight distribution or throwing off your weight in one area so you have to compensate in another area, to become stronger and more stable. Check out a few of the following examples of ways you can squeeze in a little extra core training by challenging your balance and making small adjustments throughout your day while you're at home:

✓ Blow-dry your hair standing on one leg!

✓ Lift one leg in the air and straighten your knee as you're watching television.

✓ Pretend you're tightening your belt throughout the day so you remember to suck it in.

✓ Replace your office chair with the exercise ball for at least one hour a day.

✓ Sit with crossed legs on the floor in front of the TV, or wherever else you spend a lot of time sitting, to strengthen your lower-back muscles and build a better core.

✓ Sit up tall when you're at the dinner table or anytime for that matter!

These are just a few examples of fun things you can do to start working on your core strength every day. And hopefully you'll continue to do them at home even after you've mastered the following workout.

Easing into It: Lowering to the Ground for Core Strengtheners

Revving up your circulation by increasing your blood flow to the pelvis, hips, and other parts of your body is always a good idea before launching into a series of intense crunches. The following series includes a couple of smooth moves to help you start out slowly.

Lying pelvic tilts

Pelvic tilts done lying down loosen up your hip and core area and get your circulation flowing so everything moves more freely. Take your time with this movement, and don't forget to breathe!

To do this exercise, follow these steps:

1. **Lie on your back with your knees bent and feet hip width apart. Keep your feet flat on the floor and make sure your spine is in the neutral position (see Figure 5-1a).**

2. **Keeping your back on the floor, slowly exhale as you roll your hips forward or up toward the ceiling, until your lower back is pressed flat on the floor.**

3. **Inhale as you return to the starting position, then roll your hips backward until your lower back arches slightly (see Figure 5-1b).**

4. **Repeat ten times.**

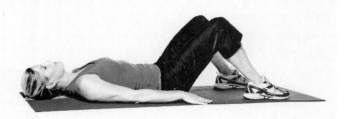

a

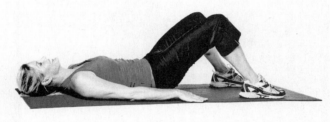

Figure 5-1:
Lying pelvic
tilts.

b

Remember the following tips for this exercise:

- ✔ Do focus on just moving your lower back and not your thighs.
- ✔ Don't tilt or hold the movement too long. Go only to the point of feeling good without straining.
- ✔ Don't hold your breath — keep your breathing steady and strong.

Hip lifts with knees together

The first exercise warmed you up so now this exercise focuses on loosening you up. For this exercise, use a smaller range of motion or don't lift your hips too high off the ground, to avoid stress on your lower back.

To do this exercise, follow these steps:

1. **Lie flat on your back, keeping your knees bent and tight together.** Place your feet flat on the floor and your arms at your sides. Keeping the spine neutral, pull your belly button in toward your spine (see Figure 5-2a).

2. **Slowly lift your hips toward the ceiling, allowing your butt and lower back to lift toward the ceiling and off the floor (see Figure 5-2b).** Hold for three to five seconds.

3. **Slowly lower your hips back down, allowing your back to return to neutral position and keeping your knees pressed tight.**

4. **Repeat ten times.**

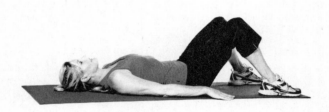

a

Figure 5-2:
Hip lifts
with knees
together.

b

While you do this exercise:

✔ Pull in your abdominal muscles, for support.

✔ Maintain a neutral spine.

✔ Don't hold your breath.

Suiting Up Your Core

Ah, the sit-up . . . now known as the crunch because, face it, people just don't like doing sit-ups. The exercise community had to come up with a new word to market these moves. However, you do crunches slightly different than sit-ups: Instead of starting the movement with your arms and trying to sit up with the strength of your upper body, suck in your gut and try the following series of fun crunches using only your abdominals.

Crunches

The simplest way to regain strength in your core and endurance is to do crunches. However, be sure to progress slowly. When you first try this exercise, place your fingertips behind your ears and you elbows bent and out to the sides. Then you can try crossing your arms in front of your chest, which adds extra weight and a degree of difficulty to this exercise.

 Variation: If the following crunch proves to be too difficult, try placing your hands palm down on the floor right next to your hips. Slide your fingertips about three inches toward your feet by using your abdominals to lift your shoulders off the ground. Hold briefly, and then return to starting position.

1. **Lie on your back, with your knees bent and fingertips behind your neck for support.**

   Your feet should be flat on the ground (see Figure 5-3a).

   Be sure to keep a space between your chin and chest as you're looking up toward the ceiling.

2. **Raise your chest until your shoulder blades lift off the floor (as shown in Figure 5-3b).**

3. **Slowly lower back to the floor.**

4. **Repeat five to ten times, gradually progressing to more repetitions when you feel comfortable.**

Follow these tips while performing this exercise:

- Don't use your hands and arms to help lift you up — use your abdominals.

- Keep your abdominals pulled in toward your spine throughout the entire movement.

- Don't raise your head and shoulders more than just off the ground.

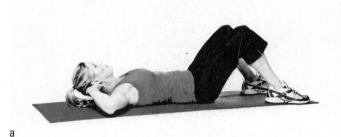

a

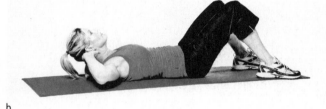

Figure 5-3:
Crunches.

b

Side crunch

The side lying crunch is a great addition to your beginner abdominal program because it also helps target the side muscles or obliques. It can feel a bit awkward to do at first but try it a few times and once you get the hang of it you'll see a smaller waist along with a stronger core!

To do this exercise, follow these steps:

1. **Lying on the floor or on a mat, bend your knees and clasp your hands behind your neck (see Figure 5-4a).**

2. **Lifting your upper torso, raise yourself slightly off the floor using your waist muscles or obliques (as shown in Figure 5-4b).** Bring your elbow toward your feet to target the waist.

3. **Return back down to the floor and repeat on other side after ten repetitions.**

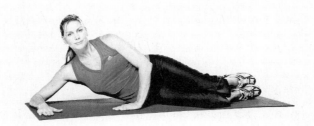

a

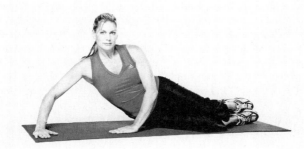

Figure 5-4:
Side crunch.

b

Follow these tips for this exercise:

- ✔ Engage your core throughout this entire exercise.
- ✔ Keep your knees on the ground and use your upper body to do the move.
- ✔ Avoid pulling on your head with your hands or it will strain your neck.
- ✔ Remember to breathe.

Side planks

The side plank strengthens the side muscles (the obliques) or waist of the body. This beginning version has you using bent knees instead of having your legs straight out to support your body weight — you can always work up to that as you gain strength in your core.

To perform a side plank, follow these steps:

1. **Lie on your left side, propping up your body on your left elbow.** Place your elbow directly beneath your shoulder. Bend both of your knees at a 90-degree angle, stacking your thighs on tops of one another (see Figure 5-5a). Place your right hand on the floor in front of your body, for support. Ensure that your body from your head down to your toes is in a straight line, with a neutral spine.

2. **Lift your hips so that your torso comes off the ground and your body is in a straight line from your head down to your knees.** If you can, take your right hand off the floor and place it alongside your body. Try to hold this position for 15 to 30 seconds (see Figure 5-5b).

3. **Repeat for three repetitions and increase reps as the exercise becomes easier.**

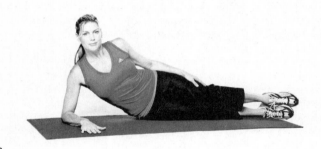

a

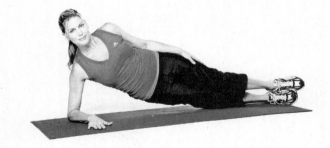

Figure 5-5:
Beginning
side plank.

b

Follow these tips for this exercise:

✔ Pull your abdominal muscles in for support.

✔ Don't allow your hips to drop down toward the ground.

✔ Don't hold your breath — keep your breathing steady and strong.

Bicycles

Hands down, this exercise is the best core exercise for targeting the waist, obliques (the muscles that run down the side of the waist), and abs. The twisting and pulling motion you do with your knees and upper body is perfect for getting your core in shape fast!

To do this exercise, follow these steps:

1. **Lie on your back with your knees bent and thighs perpendicular to the floor.** Place your fingers just behind your ears (see Figure 5-6a).

2. **Lift your shoulders off the floor as you straighten the right leg, and bring the left knee in toward your right armpit. Without relaxing the torso or returning your shoulders to the floor, repeat on the other side by straightening the left leg and pulling the right knee in toward the left armpit (as shown in Figure 5-6b).**

3. **Alternate the legs in a slow bicycling movement.**

4. **Repeat 15 times on each side.**

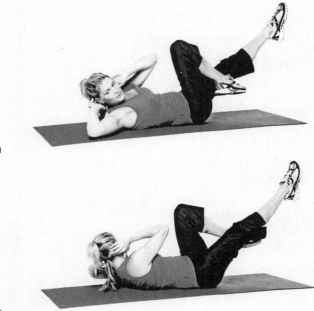

a

b

Figure 5-6:
Bicycle for the waist and abs.

Remember these tips while bicycling:

- ✔ Pull your abdominal muscles in for support.
- ✔ Don't allow your hips to drop down toward the ground.
- ✔ Don't hold your breath — keep your breathing steady and strong.

Push-ups on knees

You may be wondering what push-ups have to do with your core. After all, haven't you always been told to do push-ups to tone your upper body? Although push-ups have traditionally been the go-to exercise for upper-body toning, push-ups on your knees are a good way to regain strength in your belly and core area. When you do a push-up, you recruit your core muscles to help keep your back straight and assist you in pulling your belly button in toward your spine. You can progress to push-ups on your toes as you get stronger; however, always keep in mind that your back should remain straight and should not buckle from the weight of your body, even when supported by your knees.

Keeping your knees on the ground with a towel beneath them will ease the harshness of the floor and provide better support for your body.

To do this exercise, follow these steps:

1. **Kneel and place your hands on the floor in front of you, shoulder width apart (as shown in Figure 5-7a).**

   Make sure that your hands are directly below your shoulders on the floor.

2. **Lower your upper body toward the floor, bending your elbows out to the side (see Figure 5-7b).**

3. **Straighten your elbows and exhale as you press back up into the starting position.**

4. **Complete ten repetitions and increase the amount of repetitions once the exercise becomes easier.**

Consider some helpful hints for this exercise:

- ✔ Keep your abdominal muscles tight, to help you maintain your weight.
- ✔ Use proper breathing, inhaling as you lower and exhaling as you press back up.
- ✔ Don't arch your back. Keep it straight and in line with your head and the rest of your body.

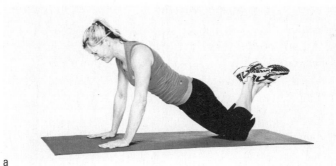

a

Figure 5-7:
Push-ups on
knees.

b

Baby Got Back!

A healthy spine is the backbone of all your core workouts (no pun intended). Gaining strength in your back muscles helps you maintain your posture and keeps you fluid with all the movements you do throughout the day. The following exercises help you gain strength in your back and tighten up your entire core so you'll notice a difference in the way you look and feel in no time.

Back extensions

The back extension exercise seems simple, yet it is a powerful and effective back strengthener. It also targets the lower back, so if you have lower back problems, you may want to skip this exercise.

To do this exercise, follow these steps:

1. **Using a mat or towel, lie on your stomach and place your arms at your sides, with the palms facing up (see Figure 5-8a).**

2. **Pulling in or contracting your abdominal muscles, lift your chest a few inches off the floor, keeping your gaze straight ahead at all times (see Figure 5-8b).**

3. **Hold for a few seconds before lowering your chest back toward the ground.**

4. **Repeat this exercise three to five times and increase reps as exercise becomes easier.**

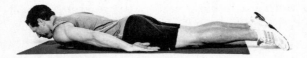

a

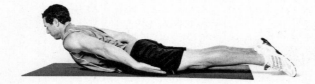

Figure 5-8:
Back
extensions.

b

Make sure you

 ✔ Tighten your butt or glutes to protect your lower back as you lift your chest off the floor.

 ✔ Tighten your abdominals throughout this move.

 ✔ Avoid lifting too high off the floor. Lift only to the point that you are not straining your back.

Plank

The plank is another top core exercise that targets the abdominals and back muscles. Stay strong and lifted during this exercise, and maintain a long, straight back.

To do this exercise, follow these steps:

1. **Lie face down, resting your forearms flat on the floor, and keep your elbows directly below your shoulders.**

   Your feet should be touching or no more than an inch apart (see Figure 5-9a).

2. **Lift your body off the floor using your forearms and toes, keeping your body as straight as possible.** Maintain this position for as long as possible, and challenge yourself as you build up to longer periods in the plank position (see Figure 5-9b).

3. **Hold the position for 10 to 15 seconds in the beginning or as long as you can before working your way up to holding the plank position for longer periods of time.**

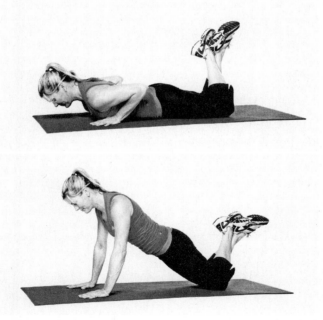

Figure 5-9:
Plank.

a

b

You don't want to forget these tips:

✔ Keep your back long and straight.

✔ Don't let your hips or knees drop toward the floor.

✔ Breathe steady and engage your abs.

Having an all-or-nothing approach to exercise: Why 20 or 30 minutes is better than trying to do 60 or 90 minutes!

My philosophy is to always start off slowly and work your way up to something — not only is it more practical but you won't get discouraged when you can't fit in 60 to 90 minute workouts and as a result decide to do nothing at all! Yes, the latest trend in exercise (which people of all demographics seem to be able to stick with) is more efficient workouts. And this lines up perfectly with what I have found to be true — "everything in moderation" . . . and I do mean everything! Keeping this in mind, the best way to accomplish your fitness goals is with shorter, more efficient workouts that provide weekly cardio and strengthening sessions. As an example, walking five days a week for 30 minutes at a time is a fantastic goal for everyone of all ages. And adding three weekly strength-training sessions of 20 minutes per session is the perfect compliment to add to your walking. Sticking to shorter walks, weekend hikes, better eating, and plenty of rest all adds up — and you usually make it home without twisting your ankle! Nice!

Chapter 6

Getting That Six-Pack: Abdominal Core Superset

In This Chapter

▶ Discovering the benefits of a superset

▶ Uncovering your six-pack

▶ Picking the best abdominal crunches for you

*B*elly fat is associated with greater health risks and lower-back pain (see Chapter 2 for more on these risks). And in this country, belly fat is far too common. America's love for fast food (or anything fast, for that matter) has caused this country to have the highest percentage of obese people in the world — and that number is still growing!

Although lower-back pain is another side effect of belly fat or weak abdominal muscles, this problem can be also be a sign of a serious medical condition. If you've been experiencing pain in your back for more than three consecutive days, see a doctor before beginning any of the exercises in this chapter.

Throughout this chapter, I give you some fantastic abdominal crunches that you can do while lying on your back or on your side. Follow the series of crunches included in this chapter and you can

✔ See that six-pack start peeking through or at least see some tone in your tummy and tightening in your waist.

✔ Build strength in the center of your body, where you need it most to help support all your movements.

✔ Build stability and create balance with all the movements you need to do throughout the day.

Shaping Up with a Superset

I mention supersets in the title of this chapter because when you're working your core, you're working opposing muscle groups and that's what you use in supersets — opposing muscle groups. So, what is a superset? Supersets are two exercises that are performed back to back or one right after the other that target opposing muscle groups. A good example of these opposing muscle groups would be the chest and back muscles that are used in many of the core exercises demonstrated in this chapter. Combining two of any of the exercises given in this chapter would create a superset. So take a look at why you "need" or should I say "want" to create a superset and go from there!

Supersets: How they are different from a regular workout

When you're performing a superset, the basic difference is that you don't rest between exercises like you would with a regular workout. In a regular workout, you rest around 90 seconds between exercises, but with a superset you immediately move from one exercise right into the next. As you move from one exercise to the next, you target two different muscle groups instead of just one that you would in your regular workout because you are performing multiple exercises within the same set — a superset!

Benefits of doing a superset

The main benefit of doing supersets is to promote small changes in your body that you may have stopped seeing. Forcing yourself day after day to do the same workout is not only boring but your body needs new challenges to promote these physiological changes. Supersets are all about learning how to push yourself into a different training zone and help excite you about working out again while increasing muscle size and conditioning.

Another benefit of doing supersets is that it cuts down your time in the gym because you're working two muscle groups within the same set. Your workouts become more efficient and more effective by performing back-to-back sets with more intensity and at a faster pace than your regular workout.

And finally, supersets are great for performing at home because you don't need heavy weights. You can push your muscles with lighter weights, which means you can get an even better workout than with heavier equipment at a gym using minimal equipment.

Shooting for a Six-Pack

Have you ever wondered if it's possible for *you* to get a six-pack? Well, you're not alone. Many people desire a great set of abs better known as a six-pack, and why wouldn't they? It not only shows hard work, but it's sexy to be able to show them off for both men and women.

However, for most of us it just doesn't come that easy and getting a six-pack means working your butt off! Genetics play a big part in how we look, and there are a lucky few who are just naturally blessed, shall we say, with a high metabolism resulting in low body fat and beautifully defined abdominal muscles. For the rest of the world though, it takes work and a few other ingredients you can find below.

What to do to get a six-pack

Here it is . . . "the secret" to getting a six-pack and guess what? It's going to take some work! Surprised? Don't be . . . anything worthwhile in life takes hard work and dedication. There are no quick fixes so read below to find the three things you can do to get washboard abs, a flat tummy, toned midsection, well, you get the point!

Low body fat

To see the muscles that make up the abdominals, you've got to reduce your belly fat. Believe it or not, you can have strong abdominals but not be able to see them because they're covered by fat. And to really see them, you have to reduce your body fat to some pretty impressive levels.

For men, your body fat level has to be at around 7 to 8 percent to see your six-pack peeking through and for women, it's 13 to 14 percent. So how do you get to those levels? Well the fastest way is to eat yourself thin with a very clean diet that is both low in fat and low in refined, processed foods. Add three days a week of strength training and up your cardio to four or five times a week and you're there! And plenty of water helps too with flushing all the toxins from your body and filling you up!

The strength training sessions should be shorter than an hour and higher in intensity (see supersets in this chapter) to keep you in the fat-burning zone. The reps you do with your exercises should be limited to 8 to 12 repetitions for maximum effect.

The best cardio to chose would be moves that are high in intensity but short in duration like running sprints. If you chose longer, more moderate intensity cardio, jogging would be good for fat burning.

Strong abdominals

Getting strong abdominals takes work but it's work you're probably already doing and you just don't realize it! Working with weights makes you use your stabilizer muscles, which are mostly located in your core (lower back and abs). And many of the weight training moves require you to transition the move through your core or midsection. See, you have the skills, you just have to up the intensity and you're on your way to that washboard stomach you've always wanted.

Detailing

Once you get your body fat down and your midsection tight and toned, you have to detail your abs, such as with spray-tanning (see the sidebar later in this chapter) to make them more visible. If you have a lot of hair on your body (men), you may need to wax, although tanning would be a less painful choice. Or you could just "manscape" which means trimming down some of your body hair to show off your new ab muscles. However you chose to cosmetically enhance your new six-pack, do it safely with products that are recommended by the dermatological association.

What not to do to get a six-pack

Any of the following techniques for getting a flatter tummy or defined six-pack are not the way to go — remember, hard work pays off and there are no short cuts:

- **Dieting to the extreme** — low-calorie diets that last more than a day or two or "fad" diets that require you to only eat one thing for more than a day are a big no-no. These diets will set you back in your quest for better abs because they cause your body to eat precious muscle that burns fat when you're body thinks you're starving. Yikes!

- **Any electric belt or devise that has to be worn around your waist** may be able to hold you together like a belt but not give you a six-pack. It may make your waist look smaller but that's about it!

- **Tons of sit-ups!** Doing 300 crunches per day will not help you get a six-pack any faster, although it may give you a stomachache! You have to simultaneously reduce your body fat and strengthen your abs to get the results you're looking for.

Crunch It! Abdominal Workout

Here it is! The series of crunches that will get you back on the path to a stronger core and a toner midsection. I suggest doing this series of crunches and abdominal exercises two to three times a week, combined with some form of cardiovascular exercise for 30 minutes five days a week.

Whether it's running in place, skipping rope, or walking at a fast pace and ending in a slow pace, be sure to heat up your core before you try the following exercises. A good warm-up will help prime your body and help you ease into exercise for a better workout.

Crunches — feet on floor

The simplest way to regain strength in your core and endurance is to do crunches. Crossing your arms in front of your chest increases the level of difficulty because it adds the weight of your upper body to the crunch.

To do this exercise, follow these steps:

1. **Lie on your back, with your knees bent, and cross your arms over your chest. Your feet should be flat on the ground (see Figure 6-1a).**

   Be sure to keep a space between your chin and chest as your eyes are gazing upward toward the ceiling.

2. **Raise your chest until your shoulder blades lift off the floor (as shown in Figure 6-1b).**

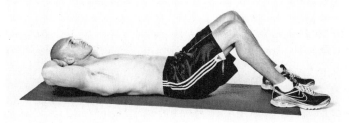

a

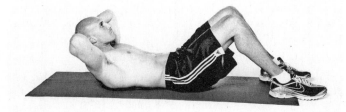

Figure 6-1: Crunches with your feet on floor.

b

3. **Slowly lower back to the floor.**

4. **Repeat five to ten times, gradually progressing to more repetitions when you feel comfortable.**

Consider these tips to get the most from this exercise:

- ✔ Use your abs, not your arms, to help lift you up.
- ✔ Keep your abdominals pulled in toward your spine throughout the entire movement.
- ✔ Keep your ribcage and lower back on the floor at all times during this exercise.

Double-crunch — knees to elbows

Just like its name, the double crunch works both the upper and lower section of the abdominals. It is an exercise that is more difficult than the basic crunch because it brings the upper body to the lower body together in a movement similar to an accordion.

To do this exercise, follow these steps:

1. **Keeping your knees bent and your feet off the floor, engage your abdominal muscles by pulling your belly button in toward your spine (see Figure 6-2a).** Place your fingertips behind your head for support.

2. **Pull your knees toward your chest, focusing on your abdominals as you bring your elbows toward your knees (see Figure 6-2b).**

3. **Slowly lower your legs and arms back to the starting position, to complete one rep.**

4. **Aim for three sets of ten repetitions.**

    Increase repetitions when you feel comfortable.

Maximize your potential for this exercise by remembering to

- ✔ Hold the movement at the top before slowly letting your knees back down toward the floor.
- ✔ Use your core muscles to control the movement.
- ✔ Let your head rest in your hands for support during the crunch — don't pull on your head with your hands.

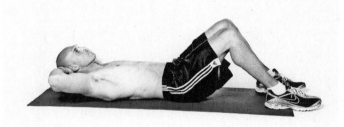

a

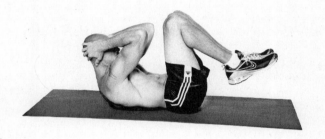

Figure 6-2:
Double-
crunch.

b

Bicycle crunches

The bicycle crunch is the best exercise to work your rectus abdominus (the ab muscle that runs right down the middle of your torso). The twisting and pulling motion you do with your knees and upper body is perfect for working the waist muscles or obliques which strengthens the sides of the body which of course, is part of the core.

To do this exercise, follow these steps:

1. **Lie on your back with your knees bent and thighs perpendicular to the floor. Place your fingers just behind your ears (see Figure 6-3a).**

2. **Lift your shoulders off the floor as you straighten the right leg and bring the left knee in toward your right armpit. Without relaxing the torso or returning your shoulders to the floor, repeat on the other side by straightening the left leg and pulling the right knee in toward the left armpit (as shown in Figure 6-3b).**

3. **Alternate the legs in a slow bicycling movement 15 times on each side.**

   Increase repetitions as you feel more comfortable with the movement.

Remember the following tips as you pedal away:

- ✔ Pull in your abdominal muscles, for support.
- ✔ Allow your hips to drop down toward the ground so you don't arch your back.
- ✔ Keep your breathing steady and strong — don't hold your breath.

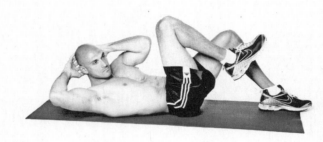

a

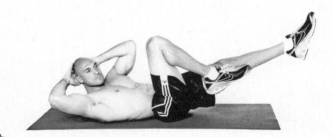

Figure 6-3:
Bicycle for
strong abs.

b

Reverse crunches

By bringing your lower body to your upper body in a reverse crunch, you target your lower abs and will see a tightening in this area faster than with other ab exercises.

To do this exercise, follow these steps:

1. **Keeping your knees bent and your feet off the floor, engage your abdominal muscles by pulling your belly button in toward your spine (see Figure 6-4a).**

2. **Pull your knees toward your chest, focusing on your abdominals as you keep your arms flat on the floor, palms facing down beside you (see Figure 6-4b).**

3. **Slowly lower your hips and legs back to the starting position, to complete one rep.**

4. **Aim for one to three sets of 10 to 15 repetitions.**

   Increase repetitions when comfortable.

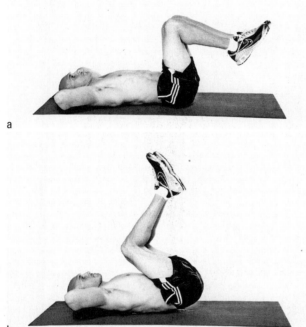

a

b

Figure 6-4:
Reverse
crunch.

Keep a couple of tips in mind:

✔ Hold the movement at the top before you slowly let your knees back down toward the floor.

✔ Keep the pace slow and steady so that you're using your core muscles to control the movement. In other words, don't go too fast!

Legs straight up crunches

You do these crunches the same way that you do a regular abdominal crunch, except that you use the added weight of your legs to increase the level of intensity for this exercise. The little bit of extra adds up to really big results! However, this is an advanced crunch and should not be done by beginners.

To do this exercise, follow these steps:

1. **Lying on your back on a mat or the floor, extend your legs straight up in the air above you. Place your hands behind your head, with your elbows out to the sides for support (see Figure 6-5a).**

2. **Keeping your elbows out to the sides, raise your head, shoulders, and upper back off the floor about three inches (see Figure 6-5b).**

3. **Hold for a few seconds before returning to the starting position.**

4. **Complete ten repetitions and increase when you feel comfortable with the movement.**

Remember to

✔ Support your head and neck with your hands.

✔ Keep your abdominals tight and engage your core.

✔ Not use your arms to pull yourself up — use your abs!

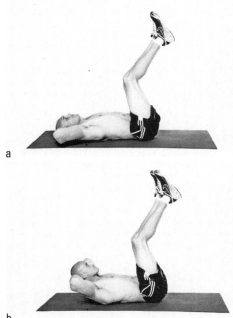

a

b

Figure 6-5:
Legs
straight up
crunches.

Side plank

The side plank strengthens the side muscles or waist of the body. Do this exercise using a mat to cushion your elbow and forearm as they support your body weight. And be sure to stack your feet on top of one another, to help hold up your body weight during this exercise.

1. **Lie on your left side, propping up your body on your left elbow. Place your elbow directly beneath your shoulder (see Figure 6-6a).**

   Place your right arm alongside your body or rest it at your side.

2. **Lift your body and hips off the ground so that your torso comes off the floor and your body is in a straight line from your head down to your feet.**

   Make sure to keep your head in neutral position to keep your spine in proper alignment.

3. **Try to hold this position for 15 to 30 seconds (see Figure 6-6b).**

4. **Repeat for three repetitions and increase repetitions when you feel comfortable.**

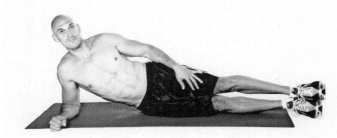

a

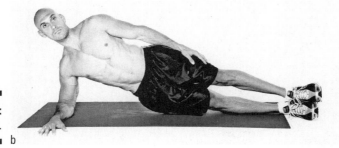

Figure 6-6:
Side plank.

b

These tips will ensure that you do this exercise correctly and safely:

- ✔ Pull in your abdominal muscles, for support.
- ✔ Don't allow your hips to drop toward the ground.
- ✔ Keep your breathing steady and strong — don't hold your breath.

Side-lying crunch

The side-lying crunch is a great addition to your abdominal program because it targets the side muscles (obliques), helping to define your waist. It can feel a bit awkward to do at first and is sometimes easier to do with the assistance of an exercise ball, but with or without the ball, it's a great core strengthener.

To do this exercise, follow these steps:

1. **Lying on the floor or on a mat, bend your knees and clasp your hands behind your neck (see Figure 6-7a).**

2. **Lifting your upper torso, raise yourself slightly off the floor using your waist muscles or obliques (as shown in Figure 6-7b). Bring your elbow toward your feet to target the waist.**

3. **Return to the floor and repeat on the other side after ten repetitions.**

    Increase repetitions as you feel comfortable.

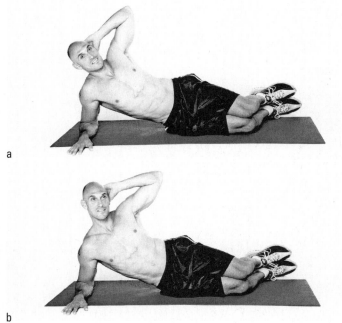

a

Figure 6-7:
Side-lying
crunch.

b

You can get the most from this exercise if you

- ✔ Engage your core throughout this entire exercise.
- ✔ Keep your knees on the ground and use your upper body to do the move.

✔ Don't pull on your head with your hands, or it will strain your neck.

✔ Breathe!

Half-up twists

Half-up twists are great for the entire core, not just the abs. The back, waist, and abdominals all get targeted with this challenging exercise. As a bonus, your butt gets a good workout too!

To do this exercise, follow these steps:

1. **Sit up tall on the floor on a mat, and put your hands on top of your knees.**

2. **Lean back until your arms are straight. Cross your arms in front of your chest, with each hand holding an elbow (see Figure 6-8a).**

3. **Twist at the waist from side to side, engaging your core as you sit up tall (as shown in Figure 6-8b).**

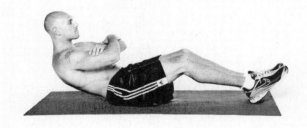

a

Figure 6-8:
Half-up
twists:
twisting
at the
waist from
side to side.

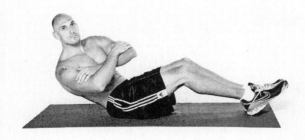

b

Follow these tips for this exercise:

✔ Let your head follow the movement from side to side with you.

> ✔ Lean back and use the strength of your abdominals to help you with this exercise.
>
> ✔ Sit up nice and tall — don't let your shoulders and back round over.

Plank leg lifts

Performing the plank with leg lifts makes for a killer core exercise. This exercise targets the abdominals and back while helping you maintain a straight, healthy spine. Be sure to stay lifted and maintain a straight back during this exercise. Great core strengthener. . . .

To do this exercise, follow these steps:

1. **Lie face down, resting your forearms flat on the floor; keep your elbows directly below your shoulders.**

   Your feet should be touching or no more than an inch apart.

2. **Lift your body off the floor using your forearms and toes, keeping your body as straight as possible (see Figure 6-9a).**

3. **Lift each leg one at a time off the floor before returning to the starting position (see Figure 6-9b).**

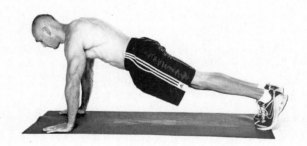

a

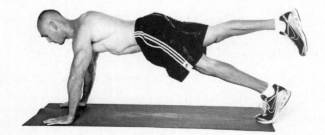

Figure 6-9:
Plank leg
lifts.

b

4. **Repeat for ten repetitions and increase repetitions when you feel comfortable.**

Maximize the benefits of this exercise by doing the following:

✔ Keep your back long and straight, in line from your head to your heels.

✔ Avoid letting your butt or hips drop toward the floor.

✔ Breathe steadily.

✔ Engage your abs and be sure to keep your leg straight and your butt contracted to help lift the leg.

Superman — opposite arm and leg extension

The Superman trains your entire core to work together properly, to provide stability and balance, while at the same time strengthening your abdominals. Remember, keeping your back strong and flexible is the best prevention against low back problems.

To do this stretch, follow these steps:

1. **Lie face down on a mat or the floor, with your arms extended overhead and palms facing down (as shown in Figure 6-10a).**

2. **At the same time, extend your right arm and your left leg out straight from your body and hold them out about three to five inches off the floor (see Figure 6-10b).**

   Imagine that strings are attached to your hand and foot, and that the strings are gently pulling your arm and leg away from each other, not up. You want to get the lengthening in your abdominal muscles and your spine, not shortening or compressing it.

3. **Hold the position for five to eight seconds, breathing comfortably and normally.**

4. **Lower your arm and leg, and return to the floor.**

5. **Repeat the exercise five or six more times on each side and increase repetitions when you feel comfortable.**

Make your Superman soar to new heights by remembering to

✔ Keep your abdominals tight. Lax abdominals may place undue stress on your lower-back muscles.

✔ Not arch your back.

✔ Not lift your foot or hand higher than 3 to 5 inches off the floor.

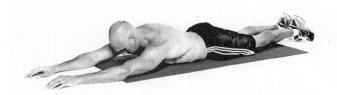

a

Figure 6-10: Lifting your opposite arm and leg in the Superman pose.

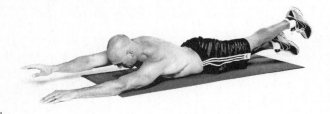

b

Spray-tanning those perfect abs

If you've seen *Dancing with the Stars* on television — and who hasn't? — you're familiar with the trick of spray-tanning! Each week the dancers get darker and darker, and look more and more sleek, don't they? Yes, a lot of it has to do with their dance training, which does work your core intensely for weeks on end, but the finishing touch is the spray tan!

Much better than going out in the sun these days, visiting a tanning salon that offers spray-tanning is the hottest trend. Although you have to stand sans bathing suit in a booth while someone of the same sex sprays you with something that looks like a blow-dryer (you can wear a bathing suit, but it does leave a stain), spray tanning is painless and super quick!

Costing anywhere from $40 to $50 a session, your new spray tan will last around ten days, depending on how often you shower or go in a hot tub. You'll want to shower first and exfoliate afterward, or wash with a loofah, before you get a spray tan so it goes on evenly and lasts longer.

For the best results, I suggest doing the workout in this chapter two to three times a week for the next month and then go for your new spray tan. You'll see a bigger difference in your tummy after you shore up your core a bit — and, believe it or not, they can actually etch a line down the middle of your rectus abdominus or midsection to make it look like you have a six-pack . . . now ain't that good news?

Chapter 7

Core Workout for a Better Butt

In This Chapter

▶ Working your core along and your lower half

▶ Getting a great butt workout

▶ Developing stronger glutes

▶ Shaping up your butt, hips, and core

▶ Getting familiar with the muscles of your lower body

▶ Loosening up your hips and buttocks

A s you age, excess weight tends to gravitate toward the lower half of the body — yep, that means your butt! By now, most of you have probably discovered this for yourself. For women, the extra pounds usually come from giving birth and for men, well, I think they call that "sympathy weight" (tee-hee). However, it's really from a lack of exercise and usually sitting around all day at work and/or watching too much television.

The large muscle groups that exist in the lower half of the body can be targeted more effectively with a tough workout, which I include in this chapter, that transitions all your rear moves through your core. So the lifting, tightening, and strengthening you'll be doing for your tush will be enhanced with a great core workout to booty, er, to boot.

In this chapter, I break down the muscles that make up your behind and get to the bottom of the best moves for your lower half, incorporating those moves into a tough workout that is sure to enhance your core assets.

The core is the bridge that connects the upper and lower half of your body. So to work your butt, you have to use your core! And vice versa. After you conquer the core moves in this chapter, try Chapter 6 for your abdominals to even things out a bit, and you'll have the best butt and tightest core on the beach!

Getting Some Junk in Your Trunk

There are three main movements you'll be using to work your lower half in the following exercises: squeezing, stretching, and stepping.

In the following list, I describe the three main movements you use to work your lower half as well as how the exercises in this chapter can give you some junk in your trunk (and that's a good thing!):

✔ **Stepping:** The *hip flexors* allow you to bend your hips and upper legs, and you use them when you step into a lunge or take one big step forward. As you do the lunge exercise or the squat, you use your hip flexors to control the movement and strengthen your hip joints as you maintain your body weight with your quadriceps and hamstrings or lower legs.

✔ **Squeezing:** Your *glutes* or butt is made up of three major muscles that work together to move your thigh away from your body or out to the side, to allow your leg to stretch out behind you and to turn your leg in and out as needed. As you lift your butt during the plank with leg lift exercises, you squeeze (or contract) your glutes to create a shapelier derriere.

✔ **Stretching:** Your *hamstrings* and *quadriceps* are the muscles that make up the upper leg, and you need to stretch these muscles so they can gain strength and provide stability throughout the lower body. As you stretch out these muscles in your legs and butt in opposite directions for the plies and side lunge, you increase the stretch in the gluteal muscles and the lower leg muscles, which creates a leaner lower body.

Breaking Down Your "Butt"

To enhance your wealth of knowledge about the butt, check out these terms regarding the hip and buttocks muscles and their functional roles and tuck these terms away (and no, "functional roles" doesn't mean ordering a shake with your fries):

✔ **Glutes:** One of the primary muscles of the buttocks, "glutes," is a slang word that collectively refers to the three muscles in the buttocks:

• **Gluteus maximus:** The largest and most superficial muscle in your buttocks, the maximus, is responsible for hip extension, and it also helps rotate the hip outward.

• **Gluteus medius:** This muscle is the middle-sized glute muscle, and its function is to move your leg to the side (abduction of your hip joint). It also helps rotate your thigh inward and outward.

> • **Gluteus minimus:** The smallest and deepest of the glutes. It also functions as a hip abductor and rotates the thigh inward and outward.

If either the gluteus maximus or minimus is excessively tight or weak, you can experience lower back pain or other postural problems. That's why it's important to balance the strength in your butt with core strength to provide stability in your body and prevent injury from muscle imbalance.

My Core Secrets Workout

The following exercises may be a pain in the rear, but (no pun intended) they'll pay off big time by giving you a leaner, toner lower body and a shapelier core.

Before you begin this workout, do five to ten minutes of cardio exercise. You can jump rope or take a brisk walk that starts at a slow pace and ends at a faster one or try the warm-up exercises in Chapter 4 of this book. A good warm-up gets your circulation going and increases the flexibility in your hip joints before you begin the following workout. Because walking is a good all-around exercise that can help alleviate built-up tension in the lower half of your body, I strongly suggest adding it at the beginning or end of this workout. You can also try doing some lower-body stretching to increase your flexibility and help your body relax after this workout if you head to Chapter 14. You'll find the butt and back stretch and a great gluteal stretch that I suggest doing to prevent any stiffness or soreness that may have accumulated in your lower half.

Squats — half up, half down

You will be doing squats in this exercise as you work your core by pulling it in tight! All the large muscle groups in the lower half of your body get a good workout in the squat — half up, half down exercise by pausing halfway down when you lower down into your squat and pausing halfway up when you raise up out of your squat to standing.

To do this exercise, follow these steps:

1. **Stand with your feet wider than shoulder width apart. Toes and knees should be pointing forward. Engage your abdominals and stand tall (see Figure 7-1a).**

2. **Slowly lower your butt halfway toward the ground and pause for a moment before lowering all the way down to a 90-degree angle in the squat position as if you were going to sit back in a chair (see Figure 7-1b).**

Keep your weight in your heels and your back as upright as possible.

3. **Exhale and tighten your abdominal muscles as you press back up into a standing position, pausing halfway for a moment, before returning to standing position.**

   Complete 10 to 15 repetitions.

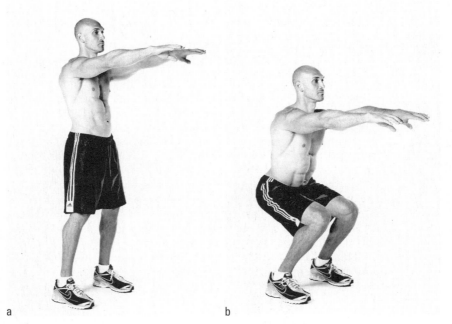

Figure 7-1:
Squats —
half up, half
down.

a   b

Remember to:

- ✔ Keep your abdominal muscles tight to protect your back while doing this exercise.

- ✔ Avoid letting your knees go beyond your toes to prevent from placing strain on your knees.

- ✔ Make sure that you don't let your butt drop down below hip level. Remember you're sitting down in a pretend chair so you won't need to press back that far.

Reverse lunges — half up, half down

This reverse lunge is a great butt and core strengthener along with giving you killer abs.

You can add weights to make this exercise more intense as shown in this exercise.

To do this exercise, follow these steps:

1. **Stand with your feet shoulder width apart.** Step or lunge back with your right leg bending your left knee at a 90-degree angle (as shown in Figure 7-2a).

2. **Push halfway through and pause for a moment before pushing straight up with your right knee as you contract your butt muscles (see Figure 7-2b).**

3. **Hold the knee raise for a few seconds before returning your leg behind you to starting position.**

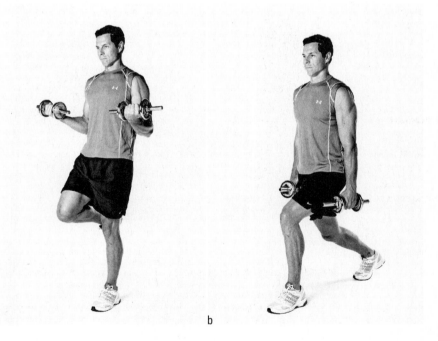

Figure 7-2:
Reverse
lunges.

a   b

Follow these important tips while doing this exercise:

✔ Keep a straight back and not an arched one.

✔ Make sure you hold for a few seconds as you raise your knee.

✔ Pull your abs in tight and contract your butt muscles before doing this exercise.

Plank leg lifts

The plank with leg lifts is a killer core exercise targeting the butt and the abdominals. Be sure to stay lifted and maintain a straight back during this exercise.

To do this exercise, follow these steps:

1. **Lie face down resting your forearms flat on the floor, keep your elbows directly below your shoulders.** Your feet should be touching or no more than an inch apart.

2. **Lift your body up off the floor using your forearms and toes, keeping your body as straight as possible (see Figure 7-3a).**

3. **Lift each leg one at a time off the floor before returning to starting position (see Figure 7-3b).** You don't have to lift the legs more than half an inch to get the benefit of this exercise.

   Repeat for ten repetitions.

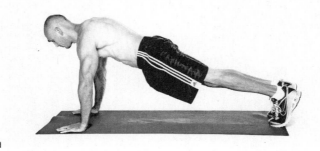

a

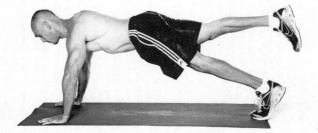

Figure 7-3:
Plank leg
lifts.

b

Here's what you need to keep in mind for this exercise:

✔ Keep your back straight and in one long line from your head to your heels.

✔ Avoid letting your butt or hips drop down toward the floor.

✔ Breathe steady and engage your abs.

Side lunge, left and right

The side lunge uses the same technique as the forward lunge only you'll be stepping step out at a 45-degree angle from the starting position instead of straight forward. It's good for strengthening your butt muscles and working your abdominals.

To do this exercise, follow these steps:

1. **Standing with your feet about shoulder width apart, keep your legs straight but not locked.**

2. **Take one large step sideways with your right leg. Slowly push back up using your right leg, butt, and core muscles to standing position (as seen in Figure 7-4).**

Alternate sides — doing ten reps on each leg.

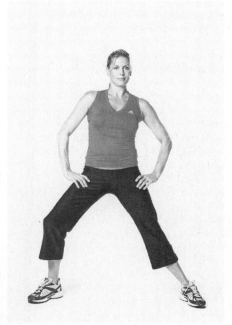

Figure 7-4:
Side lunges.

While doing this exercise, remember to

✔ Keep your hands on your hips as you step out sideways into a lunge.

✔ Keep your knees soft — don't lock your knees.

✔ Keep your breathing steady and strong — don't hold your breath.

Lunges — half up, half down

Lunges really work your butt as they call on your core muscles to help keep your chest lifted, shoulders back, and midsection strengthened. The lunge strongly defines your butt and quadricep muscles.

To do this exercise, follow these steps:

1. **Take a big step forward with your right leg and lower your right knee halfway down toward the floor. Pause for a moment before lowering down into a full lunge position with your thigh at a 90-degree angle to the floor.**

2. **Exhale as you straighten your knees halfway up to standing, pause for a moment before returning to starting position (as shown in Figure 7-5).**

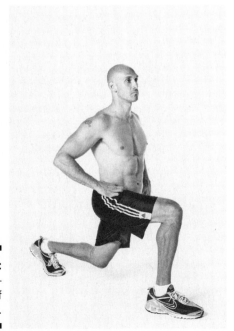

Figure 7-5:
Lunges —
half up, half
down.

You get better, safer results if you follow these tips for this exercise:

- ✔ Keep your arms close to your sides or hands on your hips while performing this exercise.

- ✔ Keep your back straight and long as you point your tailbone down towards the floor — don't arch your back.

- ✔ Keep your eyes lifted and looking straight ahead — don't let your head drop down.

Would you like to do a split?

Can you do a split or was it just never possible? Perhaps the real question is not whether you could or not but why in the heck would you even try?

To do a split it requires a lot of flexibility and technique. And if you're not performing in the Cirque du Soleil, it might not be worth the payoff. However, if doing a split is something you've always wanted to do, follow these guidelines:

- ✔ Warm up properly.

- ✔ Perform individual stretches for your hamstrings, quads, and inner thighs (see examples in Chapter 14).

- ✔ Make sure these areas are warm and limber before you make your first attempt.

- ✔ Begin kneeling on one leg, and place your opposite foot out in front of you flat on the floor.

- ✔ Slowly slide the knee beneath you backward as far as you can.

- ✔ Notice that your front leg will gradually extend. Find your comfort zone and stay there for a few deep breaths.

- ✔ Inhale, and as you exhale; see if you can move the knee back a little farther and take the stretch a little deeper.

- ✔ Hold the stretch for 30 seconds and then release the stretch by coming back to the starting position.

- ✔ Try the stretch again and repeat two or three times — each time trying to go a little deeper and getting your legs straighter.

In a perfect split, both legs must be straight, both hips facing forward, and the buttocks of your front leg on the floor. You probably won't get it the first time you try, but you can gradually get a little farther every day. Don't be discouraged and certainly don't expect to be able to do a perfect split right away! It will take weeks of slowly and progressively increasing your range of motion in the split position. As with any stretch, perform this one slowly and carefully and pay attention to form.

It's really fun to do something you thought was impossible, and many of you may think it's impossible to do a perfect split. But you never know until you try, right?

Bridge

The bridge lift combines your tush and your core as you press your hips up toward the ceiling and squeeze your butt muscles. Your hips and lower back get targeted in this exercise also.

As you lift your hips up, you need to keep your back from sagging or arching.

To do this exercise, follow these steps:

1. **Lie on the floor with your knees bent and feet flat on the floor. Rest your arms flat on the floor alongside your body (see Figure 7-6a).**

   Make sure that you keep your knees stacked over your ankles.

2. **Press your hips as high as possible toward the ceiling (see Figure 7-6b).**

3. **Slowly lower your hips down to starting position.**

   Complete 10 to 15 repetitions.

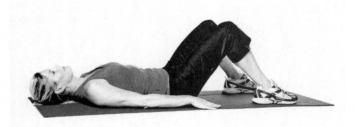

a

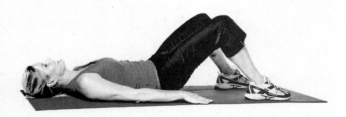

Figure 7-6:
Bridge lifts.

b

When you do bridge lifts, remember to

✔ Squeeze your buttocks tight and pull your belly button toward your spine during this exercise.

✔ Keep your lower body tight and pressed up during this exercise — don't let your hips and butt sink toward the ground.

✔ Keep your hands on your hips to help steady your body.

✔ Keep your hips even with your torso — don't press your hips too high.

Bridge with knees together

This exercise works the butt, hips, abdominals, and lower back better known as your core. Be sure to use a smaller range of motion or don't lift your hips too high off the ground to avoid stress on your lower back.

To do this exercise, follow these steps:

1. **Lie flat on your back, keeping your knees bent and tight together. Place your feet flat on the floor and your arms at your sides. Keeping the spine neutral, pull your belly button in toward your spine (see Figure 7-7a).**

2. **Slowly lift your hips up toward the ceiling, allowing your butt and lower back to lift up toward the ceiling and off of the floor (see Figure 7-7b).**

   Hold for three to five seconds.

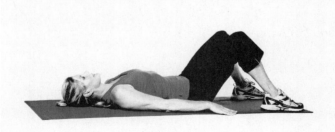

a

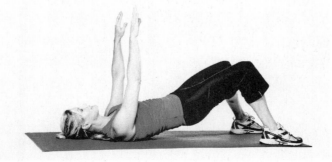

Figure 7-7:
Bridge
with knees
together.

b

3. **Slowly lower your hips back down, allowing your back to return to neutral position and keeping your knees pressed tight.**

   Repeat ten times.

Here's what you need to remember for this exercise:

- ✔ Pull your abdominal muscles in for support.
- ✔ Maintain a neutral spine.
- ✔ Breathe! Don't hold your breath.

Chapter 8

Putting It All Together

- -

In This Chapter

▶ Knowing the benefits of circuit training

▶ Understanding how little moves add up to big core changes

▶ Getting the best core exercises to do on your back and stomach

▶ Core strengthening from your head to your toes

▶ Finding out what makes up a total body workout

- -

*T*his chapter is geared toward giving you a total body workout, especially if you're short on time. When you can do this workout comfortably two or three days a week, you can start to increase your resistance by adding one of the accessories shown in Part III of this book.

However, if you want to work a particular area of the body or you want to focus on arms one day and legs the next along with your core, the specialized chapters in Part II of this book are better suited for you.

Adding cardiovascular training to go along with the total core workout is ideal. Walking is the perfect compliment to core training, believe it or not!

Warming up your body increases the temperature of your muscles, which reduces the risk of injury. For burning belly fat, studies show that walking is the number one suggested exercise. So I suggest 30 minutes of walking five days a week as the perfect complement to the total core series in this chapter. If you have a few extra minutes to spare and want a really great warm-up, head to Chapter 4.

When you begin using your new total body in one fitness program, you'll soon discover that it requires a lot of endurance. Like with any new form of exercise, avoid overtraining by resting 24 to 48 hours in between workouts.

Core Secrets to Looking Better Shirtless

For working your abs and back, otherwise known as your core, there are a few tricks that you can do to increase your success. The abdominal muscles respond pretty quickly to these body-shaping techniques so you can incorporate them in the workout in this chapter after you try them. Read on to see if they make a big difference for you and add up to big changes like they do for me:

- ✓ **Work harder by bringing your feet closer together.** By bringing your base, or in this case your feet, closer together when you're standing, sitting on a weight bench, using an exercise ball, or lying on the floor, you can intensify your workout because you've shortened your stride or base by bringing your feet closer together. Just for fun, try starting with your feet shoulder width apart and then with each repetition, move your feet just an inch or two closer to each other until your feet finally meet. This will increase the level of difficulty of the exercise gradually so you can feel the difference a little bit at a time and see what is most comfortable for you. Small modifications add up to big changes!

- ✓ **Increase the intensity by increasing the distance between the ball and your core.** If you're using an exercise ball for any of the following exercises, remember that the same rule applies; the farther away the ball is from your *core* (torso), the more difficult maintaining your balance is. For example, when you do a push-up on the ball, it's much easier when you place the ball underneath your lower legs because it's closer to your abs, hips, and glutes. To increase the difficulty, simply roll the ball out to your feet so that it's farther away from the center of your body, making maintaining your balance harder.

- ✓ **Always control the exercise and don't let it control you.** Kind of like the saying, "make sure you're walking the dog and the dog's not walking you," the same thought process applies here. With each repetition, make sure you think about the movement and the body part you're working so that you control it. Don't let the momentum of the exercise take over.

- ✓ **Contract and tighten your abs at the beginning of each exercise.** If you contract and tighten your abs each time you begin an exercise, you are using your core strength to help complete the exercise. The best way to do this is to take a big deep inhale before you start then immediately exhale your breath as you tighten your tummy and begin the exercise. It really works, so try it — and that's an order!

Where it's at: Locating your core

Working your core seems to be the new buzz-word these days. However, knowing exactly what it is and locating it can be a totally different story. So here's my explanation of what it is and where to find it in layman's terms!

Your core is made up of the deep abdominal and back muscles that work as stabilizers for the entire body. These muscles are referred to as deep muscles because you can't see them. Still, these muscles are responsible for maintaining the body's core stability.

The three muscles in the core, or midsection or trunk, of the body are the *transverse abdominus, multifidus,* and the *quadratus lumborum.* These muscles work together to protect the spine and to help with everyday or functional activities, such as lifting, throwing, bending, reaching, and running. So you can see why keeping the stabilizer muscles well conditioned is extremely important.

Core training has many benefits but the number one would be to strengthen the "bridge" that connects your upper body with your lower body ... I think that's the best way to think of it. If the bridge is weak, the cars aren't going to make it across.

To get the full benefits of working your upper and lower body along with your core, see the Chapters in Part II of this book which are designed specifically for the abs, butt, and back.

Maintaining the "S" Position or Neutral Spine

Being in *neutral* is really an active position where the lower abdominal and pelvic stabilizer muscles are activated to create a girdle of sorts for the body to protect itself from injury. So, when you hear the term *neutral spine* used in exercises, I'm referring to the neutral position of your spine.

To keep your back from arching and to practice neutral spine, try this exercise in front of a mirror:

1. **Stand facing the side as you look into a mirror.**

2. **Imagine a ruler extending down along your back from the top of your shoulders or shoulder blades to the bottom of your pelvis or hips.**

   You should be standing tall and straight with everything stacked up neatly as follows: head, shoulders, rib cage, pelvis, and legs.

You can also try this exercise by lying on the floor:

1. **Lie on the floor with your back pressed down.**

   If your back is flat, you shouldn't be able to put your hand between the floor and your back.

2. **Exhale as you bring your knees to your chest and think about the placement of your back on the floor.**

3. **Hold your knees to your chest for a few moments, and then release your legs back to the floor.**

   Notice how your back feels now. Is it pressed down, not arching? Can you feel the neutral position of your body as it relaxes on the floor but is actively pressed downward? If so, you should now be able to slip your hand under your lower back and feel the natural curve of your spine, otherwise known as maintaining neutral spine.

You will need to use neutral spine with all core exercises and any other workout that involves lying on the floor.

Total Core Workout

This workout provides crossover benefits for many of the activities you do in everyday life by mimicking the movements you use when you push, pull, kneel, or squat. In addition, these exercises help improve your overall core strength.

The first seven exercises in this section focus on core work that is done while lying on your back. Mastering proper form and remembering to use neutral spine throughout the following back series will help you see improvements faster and help you progress quicker through the program.

The last six exercises in this section —including the Superman and Plank positions — focus on working the core as you lie on your tummy. For most people, you will want to start off with one set and work your way up to additional sets after a few weeks.

If you find the following exercises challenging but are able to maintain proper form while doing them, then you're working out at the right level for you.

On your back core series

The following exercises are a combination of all the best exercises I give you in this book. They are put together in a specific sequence so you should do one right after the other, performing one set of ten repetitions of each. As you build in strength and stamina, you will progress to another set of ten and so on and so on. Be sure to listen to your body and only do as much or as little as feels right for you!

Abdominal crunch

Doing abdominal crunches not only works the abs but also strengthens the back and hips.

Make sure you keep your lower back in neutral spine when doing crunches to maintain proper form and support your lower back. If you let your lower back arch off the ground, you could strain it and pull a muscle. Not good!

To do this exercise, follow these steps:

1. **Lying on the floor, bend your knees and rest your feet flat on the floor (see Figure 8-1a).**

2. **As you tighten your abdominals and with your hands on either side of your head, slowly lift your shoulders from the floor toward your knees (see Figure 8-1b).**

3. **Hold the lift for a few seconds, and then slowly roll your shoulders back to the floor.**

   Complete ten repetitions.

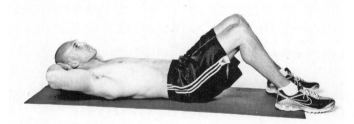

a

Figure 8-1:
Abdominal
crunch.

b

While doing the ab crunch, remember to

- Relax your neck as you curl up into a crunch.
- Keep your chin toward the ceiling and don't use your hands to pull your head off the floor.
- Maintain your neutral spine by pressing your lower back into the floor.
- Exhale as you curl up into the crunch and inhale as you release back down.

Double crunch

This exercise tightens the lower abs and upper abs by bringing the upper and lower body together like an accordion. Be sure to return to starting position each time you finish the double crunch to help you get the best toning in your midsection possible.

To do this exercise, follow these steps:

1. **Keeping your knees bent and your feet off the floor, engage your abdominal muscles by pulling your belly button in toward your spine (see Figure 8-2a).** Place your fingertips behind your head for support.

2. **Pull your knees toward your chest, focusing on your abdominals as you bring your elbows toward your knees (see Figure 8-2b).**

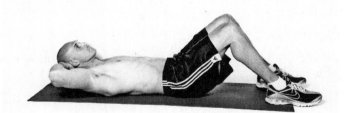

a

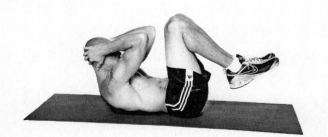

Figure 8-2:
Double
crunch.

b

3. **Slowly lower legs and arms back down to the starting position to complete one rep.** Aim for three sets of ten repetitions.

Although it sounds more like your favorite ice cream rather than your favorite exercise, you can help burn off those double-crunch calories if you remember to

✔ Hold the movement at the top before slowly letting your knees back down toward the floor

✔ Use your core muscles to control the movement.

✔ Let your head rest in your hands for support during the crunch. Don't pull on your head with your hands.

Hip lifts

This exercise works the hips, abdominals, and lower back, better known as your core. Be sure to use a smaller range of motion or don't lift your hips too high off the ground to avoid stress on your lower back.

To do this exercise, follow these steps:

1. **Lie flat on your back, keeping your knees bent and tight together. Place your feet flat on the floor and your arms at your sides. Keeping the spine neutral, pull your belly button in toward your spine (see Figure 8-3a).**

2. **Slowly lift your hips up toward the ceiling as you push through your heels, allowing your butt and lower back to lift up toward the ceiling and off of the floor (see Figure 8-3b).**

   Hold for three to five seconds.

3. **Slowly lower your hips back down, allowing your back to return to neutral position and keeping your knees pressed tight.**

   Repeat ten times.

While doing hip lifts, you need to

✔ Pull your abdominal muscles in for support.

✔ Maintain a neutral spine.

✔ Remember not to hold your breath.

✔ Avoid hyperextending your lower back.

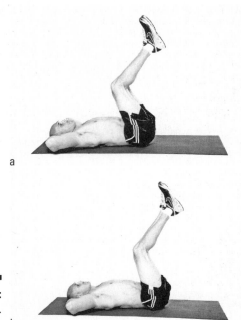

a

Figure 8-3:
Hip lifts.

b

Oblique crunches

The oblique crunch or side-lying crunch is a great addition to your core program because it targets the side muscles or obliques, helping whittle the waist.

To do this exercise, follow these steps:

1. **Lying on the floor or on a mat, bend your knees and clasp your hands behind your neck (see Figure 8-4a).**

2. **Lifting your upper torso, raise yourself slightly off the floor using your waist muscles or obliques (as shown in Figure 8-4b).** Bring your elbow toward your feet to target the waist.

3. **Return back down to the floor and repeat on other side after ten repetitions.**

For these crunches, you need to be sure to

✔ Engage your core throughout this entire exercise.

✔ Keep your knees on the ground and use your upper body to do the move.

✔ Avoid pulling on your head with your hands or it will strain your neck.

✔ Breathe!

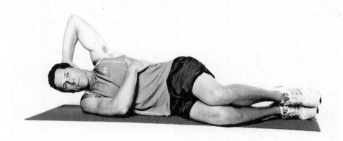

a

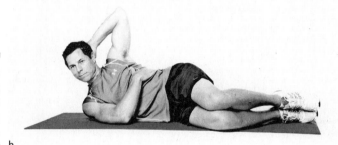

Figure 8-4:
Oblique
crunches or
side-lying
crunch.

b

Half-up twists

Half-up twists are great for the entire core and not just the abs. The back, butt, waist, and abdominals all get targeted with this challenging exercise.

To do this exercise, follow these steps:

1. **Sit up tall on the floor on a mat and put your hands on top of your knees.**

2. **Lean back until your arms are straight. Cross your arms in front of your chest with each hand holding an elbow (see Figure 8-5a).**

3. **Twist at the waist from side to side engaging your core as you sit up tall (as shown in Figure 8-5b).**

Here's what you need to remember while doing this exercise:

✔ Let your head follow the movement from side to side with you.

✔ Lean back and use the strength of your back to help you with this exercise.

✔ Sit up nice and tall. Don't let your shoulders and back round over.

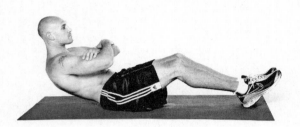

a

Figure 8-5:
Half-up
twists:
twisting at
waist from
side to side.

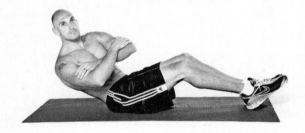

b

Bicycle crunches

This is the best exercise to work your rectus abdominus or ab muscle that runs right down the middle of your torso. The twisting and pulling motion you do with your knees and upper body is perfect for getting your core in shape fast and helps reduce your waist size too by working the obliques.

To do this exercise, follow these steps:

1. **Lie on your back with your knees bent and thighs perpendicular to the floor.** Place your fingers just behind your ears (see Figure 8-6a).

2. **Lift your shoulders off the floor as you straighten the right leg and bring the left knee in toward your right armpit.**

3. **Without relaxing the torso or returning your shoulders to the floor, repeat on the other side by straightening the left leg and pulling the right knee in toward the left armpit (as shown in Figure 8-6b).**

4. **Alternate the legs in a slow bicycling movement ten times on each side.**

Bike your way to great abs with the following tips:

✔ Pull your abdominal muscles in for support.

✔ Allow your hips to drop down toward the ground — don't arch you back.

✔ Keep your breathing steady and strong — don't hold your breath.

✔ Avoid pulling you head with your hands to avoid straining your neck.

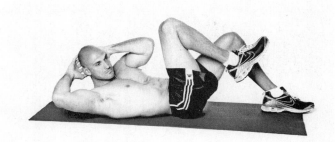

a

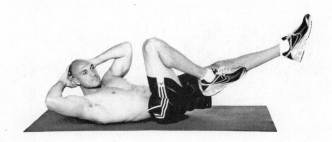

Figure 8-6:
Bicycle for
strong abs.

b

Reverse crunches

By bringing your lower body to your upper body, you target your lower abs and will see a tightening in this area faster than with other ab exercises.

To do this exercise, follow these steps:

1. **Keeping your knees bent and your feet off the floor, engage your abdominal muscles by pulling your belly button in toward your spine (see Figure 8-7a).**

2. **Pull your knees toward your chest, focusing on your abdominals as you keep your arms flat on the floor with palms facing down beside you (see Figure 8-7b).**

3. **Slowly lower hips and legs back down to the starting position to complete one rep.**

   Aim for one set of ten repetitions.

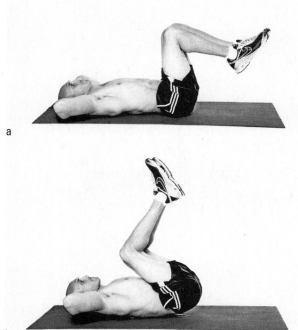

a

b

Figure 8-7:
Reverse
crunch.

Keep these tips in mind while doing a reverse crunch:

- ✔ Hold the movement at the top before slowly letting your knees back down toward the floor
- ✔ Keep the pace slow and steady so you are using your core muscles to control the movement — don't go too fast.

Half crunch

This exercise is a super strengthener for your abdominals and core muscles. It takes a lot of strength to pull your body off the ground using only your core muscles so don't let the name fool you!

To do this exercise, follow these steps:

1. **Lie on your back with your legs straight and your arms alongside your body with palms facing down.**

2. **Contracting your abs, lift your shoulders and torso off the floor first by curling up halfway, making sure to lift your head last.** Your neck should be in line with your spine (as shown in Figure 8-8).

3. **Lower back to starting position, being sure to return your head to the floor last.**

   Repeat for ten repetitions.

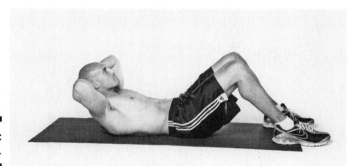

Figure 8-8:
Half crunch.

A half crunch doesn't half the work, especially when you follow proper form with these tips:

✔ Use your abdominals to pull yourself off the floor and not your hands.

✔ Exhale as you curl up and inhale as you lower back down to the floor.

✔ Keep your head in line with your spine. Don't pull on your neck muscles by lifting your neck.

On-your-tummy core series

The following core exercises are done as you're lying on your tummy. They target the abdominals and back muscles by building strength and stamina throughout your core as you hold each position.

Superman

This exercise trains your entire core to work together properly to provide stability and balance, while at the same time strengthening your back. Remember, keeping your back strong and flexible is the best prevention against low back problems.

To do this stretch, follow these steps:

1. **Lie face down on a mat or the floor with your arms extended overhead and palms facing down (as shown in Figure 8-9a).**

2. **At the same time, extend your right arm and your left leg out straight from your body and hold them out about three to five inches off the floor (see Figure 8-9b).**

3. **Hold the position for five to eight seconds, breathing comfortably and normally.**

4. **Lower your arm and leg and return to the floor.**

    Repeat the exercise five times on each side.

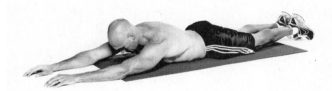

a

Figure 8-9:
Lifting your
opposite
arm and
leg in the
Superman
pose.

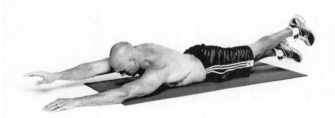

b

Work yourself super-hard with the Superman pose by remembering to

✔ Keep your abdominals tight. Lax abdominals may place undue stress on your lower back muscles.

✔ Avoid arching your back.

✔ Not lift your foot or hand higher than three to five inches off the floor.

Plank leg lifts

The plank with leg lifts is a killer core exercise targeting the abdominals and back while helping you maintain a long, healthy spine. Be sure to stay lifted and maintain a long, straight back during this exercise.

To do this exercise, follow these steps:

1. **Lie face down resting your forearms flat on the floor, keep your elbows directly below your shoulders. Your feet should be touching or no more than an inch apart.**

2. **Lift your body up off the floor using your forearms and toes, keeping your body as straight as possible. (See Figure 8-10a.)**

3. **Lift each leg one at a time off the floor before returning to starting position (see Figure 8-10b).**

   You don't have to lift the legs more than half an inch to get the benefit of this exercise.

   Repeat for ten repetitions.

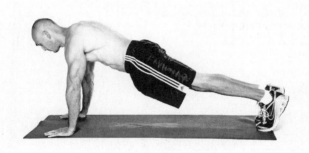

a

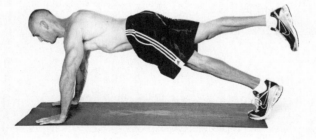

Figure 8-10:
Plank leg
lifts.

b

You can punch up the benefits of the plank if you:

✔ Keep your back long and straight in line from your head to your heels.

✔ Avoid letting your butt or hips drop down toward the floor.

✔ Breathe steady and engage your abs.

Push-ups

Push-ups target your chest and shoulder muscles along with the abdominals to give good core strength and all-over toning.

Don't let your butt dip down toward the floor during the push-up. Keep your back straight and long.

To do this exercise, follow these steps:

1. **Lie with your belly on the ground and your legs straight out behind you.** Make sure that your hands are a little wider than your shoulders on the floor (as Figure 8-11a shows).

2. **Lower toward the floor with the upper body, bending your elbows out to the side (see Figure 8-11b).**

3. **Straighten your elbows and exhale as you press back up into starting position.**

   Complete ten repetitions.

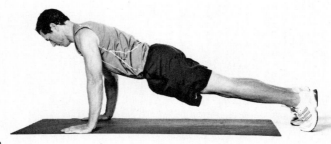

a

Figure 8-11:
Push-ups.

b

While doing a push-up:

▮ ✔ Keep your abdominal muscles tight to help you maintain your balance.

✔ Use proper breathing, inhaling as you lower and exhaling as you press back up.

✔ Keep your back straight and in line with your head and the rest of your body. Don't arch your back.

✔ Keep your elbows from locking at the top of the push-up to avoid strain on the joint.

Back extensions

Targeting the back to strengthen your abs is what core training is all about, isn't it? And the back extension exercise seems simple, yet it's a powerful and effective back strengthener. It also targets the lower back so if you have lower back problems, you may want to skip this exercise.

To do this exercise, follow these steps:

1. **Using a mat or towel, lie on your stomach, placing your arms at your sides with palms facing up (see Figure 8-12a).**

2. **Pulling in or contracting your abdominal muscles, lift your chest a few inches off the floor keeping your gaze straight ahead at all times (see Figure 8-12b).**

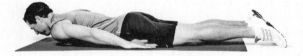

a

Figure 8-12:
Back
extensions.

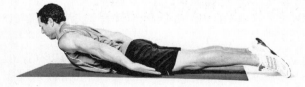

b

3. **Hold for a few seconds before lowering your chest back toward the ground.**

   Repeat this exercise three to five times.

Make the best of this back exercise by remembering to

- Tighten your butt or glutes to protect your lower back as you lift your chest off the floor.
- Tighten your abdominals throughout this move.
- Only lift to the point that you're not straining your back. Don't lift too high off the floor.

Hip extensions

This is a good strengthening exercise for the abs, glutes, and lower back. It's perfect for working on your posture and a great exercise to end your core series with!

To do this exercise, follow these steps:

1. **Kneeling on your hands and knees, place your hands below your shoulders and be sure to keep knees directly beneath your hips (see Figure 8-13a).**

2. **Raise your opposite arm and leg together off the floor, extending your leg behind you and your arm out in front of you (as seen in Figure 8-13b).** Hold for a count of three.

   Think of lengthening your body instead of just lifting your arm and leg as high as possible.

3. **Lower your arm and leg back to the starting position.**

   Repeat this exercise alternating sides for ten repetitions for each side.

Try to stay as relaxed as possible and don't tense up.

Here are a few tips to remember for this hip exercise:

- Pull your belly button toward your spine.
- Avoid tensing up your shoulders and neck.
- Keep your balance.
- Use your breath to inhale and exhale with the movement.

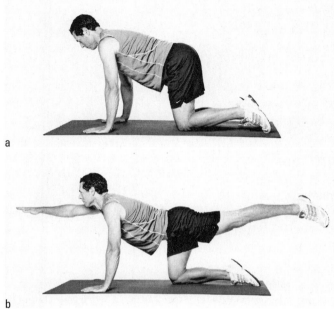

a

b

Figure 8-13: Hip extension.

Cooling Down After Heating Up

If you've ever stopped too quickly during an aerobic class or in the middle of a run, you'll know what I'm talking about — cooling down is *just as important as warming up*. Because the blood gets distributed to the extremities during your workout and needs time to return to the heart for oxygen, if you stop midstream, you can faint or get dizzy.

The best activity for cooling down your body after a workout is a five-minute, well-paced walk that ends in a slow-paced walk. Combine this with the easy core stretches in Chapter 15, and you're sure to feel relaxed and flexible when you're done with the workout in this chapter.

When you cool your body down properly by taking the time to stretch, you minimize or eliminate the muscle soreness that can result from skimping on this important step.

Circuit training

Circuit training is a fun way to train to stave off boredom and get results fast! It keeps you from burning out or getting tired of one particular exercise and challenges your body by quickly moving you through a series of exercises working different body parts at a fast pace. By moving at such a fast pace, you get the benefits of aerobic exercise in addition to the strengthening benefits you get from the series of exercises you're performing. Because circuit training is usually done in 30 minutes or less, it saves you time and burns fat more efficiently by keeping your heart rate elevated throughout the entire workout.

Switching up your workout or trying something new is a good idea when you've been consistently training in one area or training in one sport. And circuit training is a good way to try something new and exciting that can burn more fat, develop more muscles, and, of course, give you the core strength you need so badly.

Part III
Developing Core Strength Using Accessories

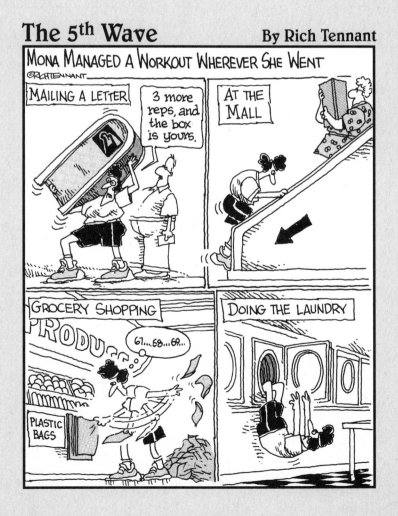

The 5th Wave   By Rich Tennant

In this part . . .

Here I give you specific core exercises to use with different pieces of fitness equipment. For instance, in Chapter 9, I give you exercises to help train your core on the exercise ball. I also show you what size ball is right for you (in case you're new to the exercise ball) and abdominal routines to help you reshape your midsection using the ball.

In Chapter 10, I give you core strength–training routines you can do with weights. I also give you complete weight-training guidelines, including how to pick the right amount of weight for you and how to choose the correct number of sets and repetitions. I even give you a little primer on weight machines and how they are used for core training in the gym. Finally, Chapter 10 shows you how to incorporate weight training into core training with upper- and lower-body exercises that are all transitioned through your core.

Chapter 9

Challenging Your Core on the Ball

● ●

In This Chapter

▶ Working your core on the ball

▶ Picking the right size ball to train your core

▶ Getting a great lesson in ball balance

▶ Developing a stronger core with the ball

▶ Shaping up your abs with ball exercises

● ●

As you get older (and, yes, we all do), excess weight tends to gravitate toward the midsection of your body, better known as your gut. For women it usually accumulates after childbirth, and for men . . . well, it usually accumulates from watching too much football and drinking too much beer. Although many different studies about how to combat slackening abdominal muscles and reducing belly fat have been done, analyzing whether cardio or weights or crunches or a combination of all is the best route, undoubtedly, no better piece of equipment can strengthen your abdominals and shore up your core faster than the exercise ball. The exercises ball challenges your balance and resistance and makes you use your internal abdominal muscles just to sit on it and keep you from falling off.

When you do the exercises in this chapter, you're bound to uncover strength that you never knew you had. The core exercises combined with the exercise ball increase your overall level of fitness and challenge your balance to help strengthen your core as you call on your deep internal stabilizing muscles.

In this chapter, I not only guide you through the proper way to choose and use your ball, but I also give you a great core workout to do on the ball. For the most efficient and effective workout, follow this workout the way I've ordered it in this chapter — don't skip around or leave anything out.

 Before you begin this chapter's workout, do five to ten minutes of cardio exercise. You can try the warm-up exercises in Chapter 4 or take a brisk walk that starts at a slow pace and ends in a faster one. After your workout, you need to stretch, to prevent any stiffness or soreness that may have accumulated in your abdominals and lower back.

Finding a Ball That Fits

You need an exercise ball to challenge your balance for the following core exercises, so you first need to know the correct size of the ball you should be using.

Using a ball that fits your particular height and weight can make or break your workout. For example, check out the possible scenarios you can encounter when using the wrong-size ball:

- If you use a ball that is too small
  - You could hurt your back because you should be sitting up tall with your thighs parallel to the floor in order to lengthen your spine and not compress it.
  - You could hurt your hips because they will sink below your knees which causes injury to the hip joint.
  - You will not be able to do the exercises properly because you will not be able to maintain a seated position.
- If you use a ball that is too big
  - You could fall off because your feet won't touch the ground when you sit on it.
  - You could have improper spinal alignment because you have to shift too much during the exercises.
  - You could hurt your hips because they should be higher than your pelvis when you sit on the ball.

The following sections give you a few great ways to pick the right ball for you. And after you find a ball that best suits you, you have to get yourself suited to your ball. I cover that next.

Sizing up the ball by using your height

When you stand next to an exercise ball, it should be even with or slightly above your knee level. Figure 9-1 provides a quick illustration. Find your height and see which ball size you should try first.

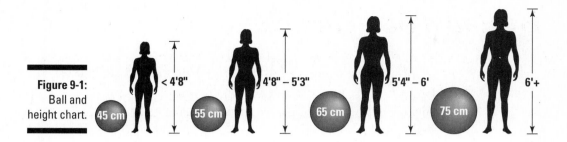

Figure 9-1:
Ball and
height chart.

The following chart shows recommended heights for the different ball sizes you can choose from.

Height	*Recommended ball size*
Under 4'8"	45 cm
4'8" to 5'3"	55 cm
5'4" to 5'10"	65 cm
5'10" to 6'4"	75 cm

For kids who are five years and younger, always use a 45 cm ball.

Sizing up the ball as if it were a chair

Another great way to tell whether your new ball is the correct height is to sit on it. When you sit on the ball, you should feel the same way you do when you sit on a chair and sit right in the middle and not off to one side. Place the ball behind you within arms reach and sit down as you guide yourself with your hands, placing them on either side of the ball. The recommended height allows you to bend your knees at a 90-degree angle when you're sitting on the ball and your feet are flat on the floor. This angle keeps your hips level with or slightly higher than your knees, with your thighs parallel to the floor.

A ball that's too small compromises the position of your hips and pelvis by lowering your hips below your knees. A ball that's too large doesn't allow your feet to touch the ground, making it unstable. Achieving a good balance between a ball that's too large and a ball that's too small gives you the best workout.

Sizing up the ball by lying on it

You can also tell if your ball is the right height by lying on it. When you lie on your stomach on the ball with your hands touching the floor and your legs extended behind you and your toes touching the floor, your back shouldn't arch and your hands should comfortably touch the floor in front of you. Your back should maintain its natural curve, otherwise known as *neutral spine* (see Chapter 4). If you arch your back at all when you lie face down with your stomach on the ball, you need to get a smaller ball, to avoid injury from placing strain on your back.

Getting a feel for sitting on the ball

When you first get your ball, sit on it with your back straight and feet flat on the floor. To get comfortable with the feel of sitting on the ball, start by sitting on it and familiarizing yourself with the sensation of contracting your abdominal muscles to keep your balance. Doing so may seem unnatural to you at first, which is perfectly normal: When was the last time you sat on a ball and not a chair? To help get the hang of it, try replacing your office chair with your ball for at least an hour a day, just to get used to pulling in your abdominals and maintaining your balance.

Finding the Perfect Spot for Exercising on the Ball

Picking the right room and the right surface for working out with an exercise ball makes all the difference in the world for your workout. You can find out more specifics in the following sections about which space is best to roll around in with your ball.

Picking the right space

The right space means finding a spot that gives you enough room to perform the exercises. Look for a space that allows you to move in any direction and stretch out properly on the floor. Keep the following in mind as you try out each space:

✔ Because you never know what direction the ball will roll or what position you'll be using with any given exercise, be sure that you have enough room to lie flat on the floor with your arms extended over your head while holding the ball.

✔ You'll also be standing with the ball above your head for some of the exercises, so make sure the space is tall enough to accommodate the ball when you're standing with it over your head.

If you're using a room in your house, find an open area or clear one that's at least 5 feet by 5 feet or 6 feet by 6 feet (if you're taller than 5 feet, 8 inches). The general rule is 2 feet longer than your height and 2 feet wider than the width of your arms. (If you lie down and pretend you're making a snow angel, you can measure the space you need that way.)

Don't forget to remove anything with sharp edges from this space, such as a coffee table or stereo, to keep from running or rolling into it when you exercise.

Searching for the best surface

It can be intimidating enough for newcomers to use an exercise ball but then to have to worry about the right surface — well that seems like a lot to worry about doesn't it? However, using the exercise ball on a hard, flat surface that you find in your house or garage works best to prevent injury. Because many of the ball exercises require you to use a non-slip surface, sticking to a hardwood surface or something that is non-skid works best.

When it comes to doing positions that require you to lie on your tummy on the ball, you'll need to place a mat underneath the ball to cushion your knees. You'll also be using the resistance of the floor in many of the exercises to keep your hands and feet from slipping.

If you have carpeted floors, you should do the ball exercises directly on the carpet because placing a mat or towel underneath the ball will make you slip. You'll also want to wear tennis shoes so when your feet come in contact with the floor they are skid proof! You can also try pushing the ball up against the couch or other heavy object in the room to prevent you from slipping and help keep your balance.

The Big Easy Core Ball Workout

The following exercises may be difficult at first because you'll have the added challenge of using the ball, but, ultimately, they'll pay off big time by giving you a tauter midsection and a toner waist.

Bridge pose

The bridge pose is a great basic exercise to increase the amount of weight you put on your abdominals, hips, and lower back.

As you lift your hips, keep your back from sagging or arching.

To do this exercise, follow these steps:

1. **Rest your head and shoulders on the ball and bend your knees at a 90-degree angle (see Figure 9-2a).**

   Keep your knees stacked over your ankles.

2. **Press your hips as high as possible toward the ceiling without allowing the lower back to arch (see Figure 9-2b).**

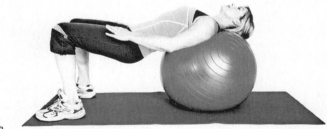

a

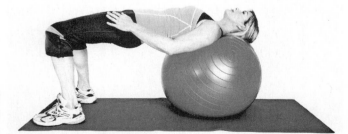

Figure 9-2: Bridge pose.

b

   3. **Slowly lower your hips to starting position.**

      Complete 10 to 15 repetitions.

While doing this exercise, remember to:

   ✔ Rest the back of your head on the ball during this exercise.

   ✔ Keep your lower body tight and pressed up during this exercise.

Bridge lift with calves on ball — straight legs

The bridge lift works your entire core area. Because you have to use your lower legs to control the movement of the ball, this exercise may also challenge your calf muscles.

To do this exercise, follow these steps:

   1. **Lie on the floor with your feet on top of the ball (see Figure 9-3a).**

      Place your arms on the floor alongside your body for support. Be sure to keep your knees slightly bent to keep tension on the muscles and not the ligaments of the knee.

   2. **Exhale as you raise your hips and pelvis toward the ceiling, pressing down into the ball with your feet to maintain your balance, keeping knees very slightly bent (see Figure 9-3b).**

   3. **Inhale as you slowly lower your hips back toward the floor.**

      Complete ten repetitions.

To maximize results with this exercise, you should:

   ✔ Keep your feet relaxed when they're resting on the ball.

   ✔ Keep your toes pointing straight up toward the ceiling and not out to the side.

   ✔ Lift your hips straight up toward the ceiling and keep a straight back.

   ✔ Keep your chin tucked into your chest — *don't* lift your chin.

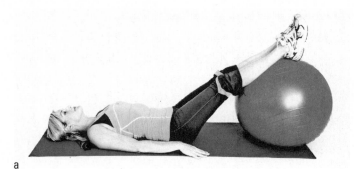

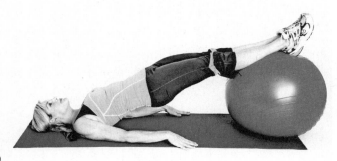

Figure 9-3:
Bridge lift
with calves
on ball.

Ball push-ups

Floor push-ups on the ball target your abdominal muscles and lower back to keep you steady on the ball.

Keeping your lower legs or shins on the ball helps you balance yourself during the push-up.

To do this exercise, follow these steps:

1. **Lie with your belly on the ball and walk your hands forward until the ball rests under your legs (as Figure 9-4a).**

   Keep your hands directly below your shoulders.

2. **Lower your upper body toward the floor, bending the elbows out to the sides (see Figure 9-4b).**

3. **Straighten your elbows and exhale as you press back up into starting position.**

   Complete ten repetitions.

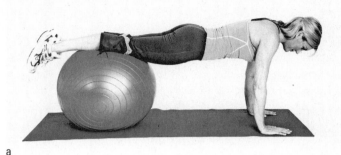

a

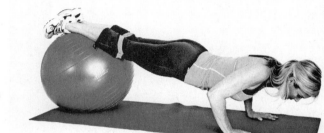

Figure 9-4:
Ball
push-up.

b

Ball push-ups work your core as long as you:

- ✔ Keep your abdominal muscles tight to help you maintain your balance.

- ✔ Use proper breathing, inhaling as you slowly lower your body and exhaling as you press your body back up.

- ✔ Keep your back straight and in line with your head and the rest of your body. Don't arch your back.

- ✔ Keep elbows slightly bent and not locked in the "up" position.

Core leg lifts

The lifting motion of your midsection used in this exercise helps create toner abs and a stronger back as well as the hamstrings and glutes. By adding the extra weight of your leg as you lift it off the ball, you'll feel a strengthening in your back muscles as well.

To do this exercise, follow these steps:

1. **As you lie on the floor, place your left leg on the ball and extend your right leg toward the ceiling (as Figure 9-5a shows).**

2. **Keeping your shoulders on the floor, lift your hips and extend your leg straight above you (see Figure 9-5b).**

3. **Point your toe and use your leg to make five small circles to the right, and then five small circles to the left.**

4. **Lower your leg back to the ball and return your hips to the floor.**

5. **Repeat this movement on the other side.**

   Complete five sets on each side.

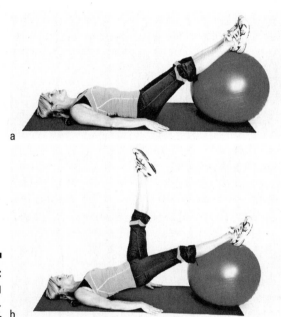

a

Figure 9-5:
Core leg
lifts.

b

When doing this exercise:

✔ Keep your arms flat on the floor alongside your body for support.

✔ Contract your abs before you lift your hips off the floor.

✔ Make sure that you don't tense your neck and shoulders as you lift your leg off the ball.

Muscles (not just cardio) burn fat!

Using different forms of resistance, such as hand weights and dumbbells, to reduce overall body fat has gotten a lot of attention lately. (I guess you cardio junkies need to take a break and read up on just a few of the reasons why a weight-training session burns more calories.)

Here are a few of the many benefits you get from resistance training:

✔ You burn 30 to 50 calories per day for each pound of muscle you put on.

✔ Building bigger muscles boosts your metabolic rate (the rate at which you burn calories) and reduces overall body fat.

✔ "Burn calories while you sleep?" Yes, it's true — lean body mass burns more calories than fat does. So if you have more muscle, you can burn more calories while you sleep.

✔ Strengthening your back muscles improves your posture and helps develop a long spine.

✔ Weight training increases your strength and muscle mass, as well as bone density, which reduces the risk of osteoporosis.

✔ Regularly working out with weights protects your joints and muscles from deterioration.

✔ Weight training strengthens the connective tissue within your body.

To burn the most calories in the shortest amount of time, you need to work the larger muscle groups in your body. Next time you're doing a workout, try a few of these compound exercises instead of exercises that target individual muscles:

✔ Squats

✔ Lat pulls

✔ Chest presses

Single-leg bridge

The single-leg bridge is a variation of the classic bridge exercise and is a much more advanced exercise. But the single-leg bridge targets your lower back, abdominals, and hips, which gives you a stronger core and hips. The single-leg bridge uses only one leg to support the weight of your entire body, so your all-important core (abs and butt muscles) gets a good workout.

To do this exercise, follow these steps:

1. **Sit tall on the ball and roll down slowly until only your shoulders touch the ball.**

2. **As you contract your abs, place your left leg across your right thigh (see Figure 9-6a).**

3. **Lift your hips toward the ceiling as you contract your butt muscles (see Figure 9-6b).**

4. **Pause for a moment and then lower your hips.**

   Complete ten repetitions before you switch legs and repeat on the other side.

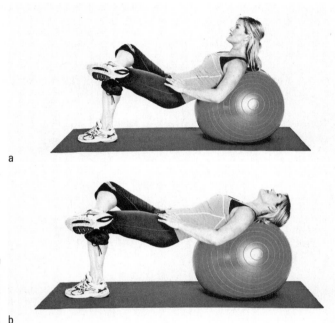

a

b

Figure 9-6:
Single-leg
bridge.

When you do a single-leg bridge, remember to:

✔ Keep your hands on your hips to help steady your body.

✔ Keep your hips even with your torso — don't press your hips too high.

Core extension

In this exercise, extending your leg behind you and placing your hips over the ball works your abs, your butt, and your back muscles to support your body and help you stay lifted.

Because you kneel on the floor in this exercise, you may want to place a floor mat or towel under your knees for comfort.

To do this exercise, follow these steps:

1. **Kneel with your chest on the ball and tighten your abdominal muscles by pulling your belly button in toward your spine.**

   Your hands should be resting on the ball for support.

2. **Extend your right leg and left arm slowly until they're opposite each other (as Figure 9-7 shows).**

   Keep your right hand resting on the ball for support. Be sure you keep your back straight and in line with your arms and legs.

   You should be able to draw an imaginary line down the center of your body.

3. **Point your toe and hold that pose for a few seconds before you return to your starting position.**

   Complete five extensions on each side.

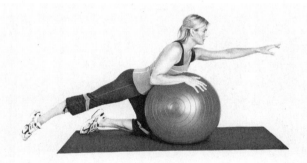

Figure 9-7:
Core
extension.

Follow these tips while performing this exercise:

- ✔ Keep your spine including your neck, on the same plane or level with your raised arm and leg. In other words, look straight down at the floor.
- ✔ Avoid arching your back when you extend your arm and leg out over the ball.

Core flexion

Your core gets a great strengthening workout with this exercise by pulling the ball into your body. As a result, you strengthen your entire lower body with this slightly more advanced movement due to the amount of balance and stabilization required by your core and shoulder muscles.

TIP

Be sure you use your core instead of your legs to pull in the ball.

To do this exercise, follow these steps:

1. **Lie with the ball under your stomach and roll forward until the ball rests under your shins (as Figure 9-8a shows).**

2. **Pull the ball in using your hips, and slowly bring your knees into your chest (see Figure 9-8b).**

   The top of your head should relax toward the floor and be in line with your spine.

3. **Hold this position for a few seconds and then slowly extend your legs back into the starting position.**

   Complete ten repetitions.

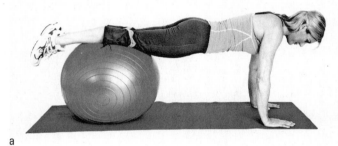

a

Figure 9-8:
Core flexion.

b

You can kick butt with core flexion if you remember to:

✓ Use your hips to roll the ball toward your chest.

✓ Make sure that you don't arch your lower back during this exercise.

✓ Keep your gaze toward the floor — don't hyperextend your neck by looking up.

Hitting Crunch Time

The best way to get killer abs is to use the exercise ball because its round shape helps place extra emphasis on the abdominal muscles. Throughout the following core exercises, your body calls upon the stabilizing muscles or core muscles to support your weight on the ball, increasing the challenge and benefits.

Traditional abdominal crunches work the outer muscles known as the *rectus abdominus.* Working these muscles in conjunction with the deeper abdominal muscles or the transverse abdominus is the best way to target the entire core of the body.

Sit-ups

Perhaps the number-one exercise used on the ball is the abdominal crunch or sit-up. This abdominal exercise is harder than traditional on-the-floor sit-ups because it requires more endurance — it's sure to kick your butt!

To do this exercise, follow these steps:

1. **Lie with the ball supporting your lower back and pelvis, Place your feet shoulder width apart and keep your knees at a 90-degree angle.**

2. **With your hands behind your head and your elbows bent out to the sides, curl your body up halfway between a sitting and a lying position (as Figure 9-9 shows).**

   Keep your tailbone pressed down on the ball.

3. ***Slowly* roll back onto the ball, one vertebra at a time.**

   Complete two sets of 10 to 15 repetitions.

You can't slack off with sit-ups as long as you:

- Draw your navel toward your spine when you contract your abdominal muscles to curl up.

- Exhale as you lift.

- Curl up and roll back down one vertebra at a time to keep from straining your back.

- Keep your gaze upward as you curl up to keep your neck in line with your spine — don't pull on your neck with your hands or allow your chin to touch your chest.

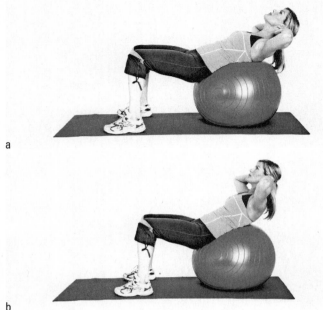

a

Figure 9-9:
Sit-ups on
the ball.

b

Oblique crunches

The oblique crunch works the muscles that run along the waist, from the pelvis to the ribcage, otherwise known as the obliques. This exercise is great for men and women who want to strengthen the muscles that define their waistlines, which will help them lose their love handles as they shore up their core.

To do this exercise, follow these steps:

1. **Kneeling on the floor, position your left hip and side of your body against the ball as you place your left arm on the ball for support. Straighten your right leg out to the side and bring your right arm behind your head so your hand is touching the back of your head (as shown in Figure 9-10a).**

2. **Crunch up, bringing your right shoulder and elbow down toward your rib cage and right leg as you exhale (refer to Figure 9-10b).**

   Keep your left hip and side against the ball at all times, to keep from slipping.

3. **Lower back down toward the ball as you slowly inhale.**

   Complete ten side crunches or oblique crunches before switching sides.

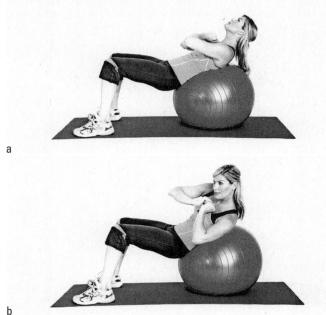

a

Figure 9-10:
Oblique
crunches.

b

Avoid injury and see results by keeping the following tips in mind:

- Keep the foot on your extended leg flat on the floor at all times for balance.

- Place your foot on your extended leg against a wall if you find yourself slipping.

- Remember to exhale as you crunch up, bringing your elbow down toward your knee.

- Don't use your hand to pull your head toward your shoulder.

Rollaways

Perhaps the second-most popular exercise for working the core area is the rollaway. This exercise is a great way to target your abs from the inside out.

To do this exercise, follow these steps:

1. **Kneeling in front of the ball, place your hands on the ball at arm's length (see Figure 9-11a).**

2. **As you contract your abdominal muscles and tuck in your butt, roll the ball away from you slightly so that your forearms rest on the ball (see Figure 9-11b).**

3. **Keeping your butt tucked in and your back straight, hold this movement for a few seconds before you return to starting position.**

   To increase the challenge, roll the ball away from you a little farther. You can also try rolling the ball slightly from side to side.

   Complete one set of 15 repetitions.

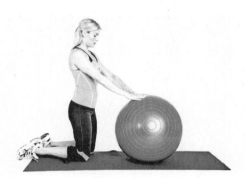

a

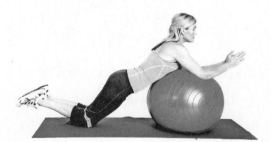

Figure 9-11:
Rollaway.

b

Make sure you do the following to get the most out of this exercise:

✔ Kneel on a cushion or mat if your knees start hurting.

✔ Keep your back long and straight to keep it from arching.

✔ Simply roll the ball out and back without holding in between. Don't hold the movement for a few seconds when the ball is rolled out in front of you, if you find this exercise too challenging.

Abdominal curls

Doing abdominal curls with the ball places the emphasis directly on the core-stabilizing muscles. By grasping the ball under your knees, the larger abdominal muscles, or outer abdominals, get used a lot more intensely during this exercise.

To do this exercise, follow these steps:

1. **Lying on the floor, rest your lower legs on the ball at a 90-degree angle (see Figure 9-12a).**

2. **As you tighten your abdominals, grasp the ball between your legs and pull toward you, lifting the ball from the floor.**

3. **With your hands on either side of your head, slowly lift your shoulders from the floor toward your knees (see Figure 9-12b).**

4. **Hold the lift for a few seconds, and then slowly roll your shoulders back to the floor.**

   Complete ten repetitions.

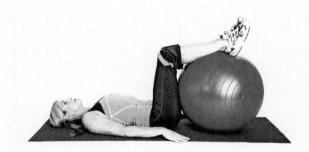

a

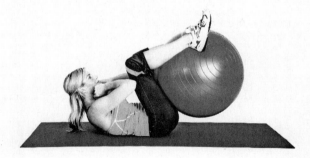

Figure 9-12:
Abdominal
curl.

b

Don't forget to do the following while performing this exercise:

✔ Relax your neck as you curl up into a crunch.

✔ Don't pull your head up with your hands to keep your head and neck in neutral alignment.

✔ Remember to exhale as you curl up and inhale as you release back down.

Ball exchange

This exercise is my favorite one for training your core. It's also good for teaching hand and eye coordination, as you'll see when you start passing the ball back and forth between your arms and legs.

This is a more advanced movement and should only be done if the abs are strong enough to keep the back from arching when lowering the ball with your legs.

To do this exercise, follow these steps:

1. **Lie on your back, making sure your lower back is pressed down. Holding the ball, extend your arms and the ball directly above your head on the floor (see Figure 9-13a).**

2. **Raise your arms and legs up to meet at a 90-degree angle above your torso (as shown in Figure 9-13b).**

3. **Exchange the ball by grasping it between your legs; then bring the ball back down to the floor (see Figure 9-13c).**

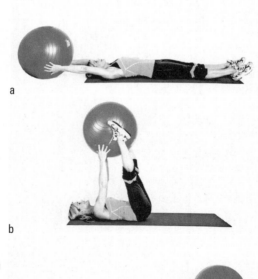

a

b

Figure 9-13:
Ball
exchange.

c

Continue exchanging the ball 10 to 12 times.

Follow these tips for this exercise:

- ✔ Avoid arching your back.
- ✔ Remember to keep a tight grip on the ball as you pass it back and forth or exchange it.

Good nutritional choices and portions for nixing belly fat!

For faster results and to enhance your core training, start adding some of the following food choices into your everyday eating plan. Of course, eating right and exercising go hand in hand, so to start getting rid of that belly fat fast, try eating a variety of foods from the following list. You'll see what a difference it makes in your waistline:

1 egg (75 calories)

1 slice whole-wheat toast (100 calories)

1 ounce cheese (100 calories)

1 apple (90 calories)

4 ounces skinless chicken breast (150 calories)

$^1/_2$ cup cooked veggies (50 calories)

1 cup green salad (100 calories)

1 cup fruit/cantaloupe (60 calories)

4 ounces salmon (175 calories)

$^3/_4$ cups pasta (200 calories)

$^1/_2$ cup cooked veggies (50 calories)

1 cup green salad (100 calories)

5 whole-wheat crackers (100 calories)

$^1/_2$ tablespoon peanut butter (50 calories)

Chapter 10

Adding Weights for Core Strength

*I*n this chapter I cover weight training to help strengthen your core. Which means, you're going to learn how to use free weights or dumbbells to combine exercises to work your core — like a squat to overhead press or a reverse lunge using weights with a leg lift. By combining two different movements, you are forced to transition the exercise through your core, so your core muscles become stronger and in turn, you are able to maintain good posture and alignment throughout the exercise. The end result is a stronger core that helps mimic the movements you use in everyday life while creating better posture and increasing stability and balance.

The best way to build strength in any part of your body is with resistance training — and using weights is the preferred form of resistance to use.

Transitioning any movement you're doing with weights through your core is what builds core strength. It also helps build functional strength, which is what you use throughout each day to reach, bend, grab, pull, and so on.

Weight training can also help reshape your body in addition to adding muscle and tone to areas that perhaps are too flat (your butt), and add definition to muscles that are just too round (your arms). If any of these body types or scenarios sound familiar to you — not to worry! Using weights works — and works fast! Within a few short weeks you will begin to see tighter, tone muscles peeking through and legs like a racehorse appearing. Well, maybe not to that extreme, but you get the point. You will see changes by adding a bit of muscle all over and reducing your body fat with weight training. So get started!

Weight Guidelines

First of all let me give you a quick overview of free weights versus dumbbells. Free weights or dumbbells are hand weights or weights that you hold in your hands (duh), that have a set weight. Whether it's 5, 10, or 15 pounds — with free weights, that's all you get. Barbells, on the other hand (no pun intended), have straight metal bars that you can add plate weights too or what is called changeable plates. Because they have changeable plates, they're good for quickly adding weight to your workout on one device rather than having five different pairs of free weights lying around. Well, now that you've had a crash course in weights, how much weight should you actually be using? Read on to find out more about the perfect weight for you!

Picking the right amount of weight for you

How much weight you use makes a big difference in the effectiveness and the success of your workout. It's always smart to choose an amount of weight that you can complete 10 to 12 repetitions with making the last two difficult, if not impossible, to complete.

Importance of increasing repetitions and sets

Instead of increasing the amount of weight you use, to challenge your body and create change, you can simply increase the amount of repetitions you do or add another set. I usually suggest starting off with one set of ten repetitions using the recommended amount of weight. That allows you to practice using good form and see where you're at in terms of evaluating your level of difficulty. After a few weeks, you should be adding at least one more set. The body adapts quickly to any amount of weight you exercise with so you have to keep up!

Plopping Down on a Weight Bench or Having a Ball

This is where my bias comes in since I am the author of *Exercise Balls For Dummies* ([Wiley] I'm never one to shy away from a shameless plug!). But there is a really big difference between using a weight bench to lift weights with or choosing to sit on an exercise ball.

When you sit on an exercise ball to do biceps curls, lat raises, T-raises or any of the other exercises in this chapter, you engage your core! Because if you didn't, you'd fall right off the ball. Now that's what I call immediate biofeedback.

Put simply, because the ball is round, it requires you to work on your balance and stability as you work other parts of your body. I prefer using an exercise ball for any kind of weight training as opposed to sitting on a bench because sitting on a chair or bench doesn't require you to pull in your abdominal muscles and engage your core. In fact, many people tend to round their shoulders and their back while using a weight bench.

So the next time you're at the gym and see one of those big round things lying around, try it out! Just make sure you keep your feet flat on the floor at all times just as if you were sitting in a chair — only better.

Dumbbell Workout for a Flat Tummy and Tiny Waist

The following exercises are challenging and fun to do. Many of them involve doing compound movements which means they combine two exercises and use two major muscle groups at one time.

Be sure to work up slowly and only do as much and as many of the exercises that you can do while using proper form.

The wood chop

The wood chop is called just that because its similar to the move you use when you're chopping wood. It's the king of all core with weight-strengthening exercises and functional stretches because it works your back, butt, abs, and chest all at the same time.

To do this exercise, follow these steps:

1. **Stand up tall with your feet hip-width apart and hold a weight in both of your hands. Bending at your waist so your upper body is parallel to the floor, hold the weight to the right side of your body (as shown in Figure 10-1a).**

2. **Sweep your arms upward and across your body so you end up with your arms over your left shoulder (see Figure 10-1b).**

   Lift from your core and hold for a breath at the top of the movement.

3. **Come back to starting position, and continue the wood chop for five repetitions before switching sides.**

To protect your back and spine, your hips should move with you and not remain forward throughout the moves.

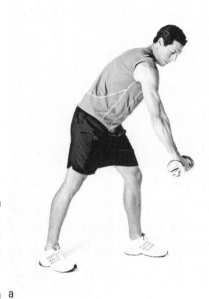
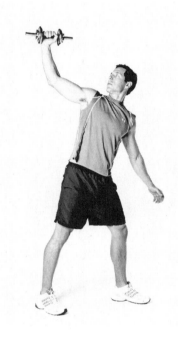

Figure 10-1:
An example of how to do the wood chop.

a   b

Remember these tips so that you don't take shortcuts with the wood chop:

✔ Inhale as you reach up and exhale as you bring your arms back down.

✔ Hold your abdominals tight to protect your back.

✔ Avoid arching or compressing your lower back.

✔ Keep the movement fluid and under control. Don't swing or create too much momentum.

Dumbbell bent-over row

This exercise transitions the movement through your core to help strengthen your back. You'll want to be sure to tighten your abdominals before performing this movement with your weight to protect your lower back.

To do this exercise, follow these steps:

1. **Holding your weight in your left hand, place your right foot in front of your left, bend at the waist so your upper body is parallel to the floor (see Figure 10-2a).**

2. **Pull the dumbbell toward your chest until your elbow is past your rib-cage and squeeze your shoulder blade back toward your spine so the muscles in your upper back are contracted (as shown in Figure 10-2b).**

3. **Lower your weight back down to starting position before continuing the next repetition.**

   Repeat for five repetitions before switching sides.

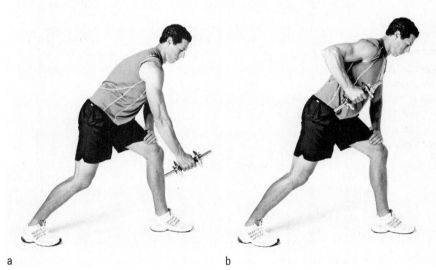

Figure 10-2:
Dumbbell
bent-over
rows.

a   b

Here's what you should remember for this exercise:

✔ Contract your abs throughout the exercise to engage your core and protect your back.

✔ Make sure your knees are bent slightly and not locked.

✔ Avoid lifting the weight past your waist.

Do's and don'ts of beating stress...

Exercise can cut your stress level in half and lower your blood pressure, which isn't a bad combination. Here are a few tips you can use to help you get back on track or just to encourage you to slow down a little:

✔ Do yoga, Pilates, or take the time to stretch to ease your body of aches and rid you of tension. Plus, it may even help you take a few much-needed breaths.

✔ Do something you love everyday. Whether it's biking, walking, playing with the kids, being active while doing something you love is the best stress reducer of all.

✔ Do realize that stress is cumulative . . . and reevaluating where you are in your life and making small changes along the way can really make a difference that shows up on a daily basis.

✔ Do think about working from home like me! With all the technology, most people can control their schedules and work from home nowadays. Taking on less of a work load, delegating chores to a relative or family member, or even moving to a smaller, tight-knit community may help you get back the simplicity you need in life to maintain a good, long, healthy life.

✔ Don't stress about stressing! Everybody is pretty much in the same boat when it comes to worrying about the everyday mundane things like work and paying bills. Be thankful for the things you do have and try not to worry about the things you don't!

Crunches with weights

This is your standard abdominal crunch but with added weight for additional strengthening of the core muscles. It can be challenging so start out slowly...

1. **Lie on your back and place your legs slightly wider than shoulder width apart. Hold weights in both your hands in front of your chest (as seen in Figure 10-3a).**

2. **Contract your stomach muscles before bringing your shoulders and upper body off the floor and toward your knees (as shown in Figure 10-3b).**

3. **Slowly return your back down to the floor before starting the next repetition.**

When doing crunches with weights, you get the most effective workout by remembering to:

✔ Hold the position for a moment before returning back down to the floor.

✔ Squeeze the weights into your chest to help keep them steady throughout the crunch.

✔ Avoid allowing the bottom of your feet to come off the floor.

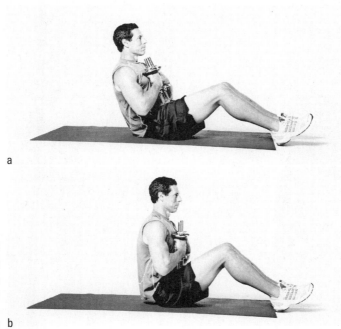

a

Figure 10-3:
Crunches
with
weights.

b

Dead lifts

This exercises strengthens the lower back and entire core as well as the legs. You will feel this exercise in your lower body also from the additional weight you'll be using as you lift up through your core.

To do this exercise, follow these steps:

1. **Taking a shoulder-wide stance, start with the weights on the floor in front of you.**

2. **Squat down to pick the weights up in front of you on the floor, being sure to keep a straight back (see Figure 10-4a).**

3. **Press through your heels to come back to standing position keeping your arms straight down at your sides and elbows straight. Pull your**

shoulders back by squeezing your shoulder blades together as you
come back to starting position (see Figure 10-4b).

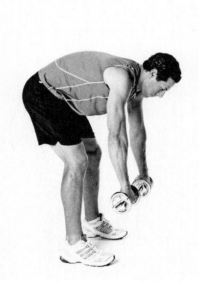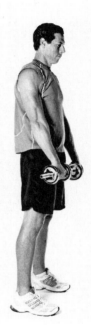

Figure 10-4:
Dead lifts.

a   b

To keep from killing yourself, use the following tips on proper form while
doing dead lifts:

- Grip the weights using palms facing down or using an overhand grip.
- Keep your arms straight throughout this exercise.
- Keep a straight back during this exercise and chin up! Don't let your
  back round.

T-Raises

This exercise requires you to lift your arms while holding weights straight
up directly through the core of your body. It's great for arms, shoulders, and
upper back as well.

To do this exercise, follow these steps:

1. **Standing tall and holding weights down at your sides, slowly raise your weights until they are straight out in front of you at chest level (as shown in Figure 10-5a).**

2. **Then like an airplane or a "T," move arms out to either side of your body (see Figure 10-5b).**

3. **Return to starting position by bringing your arms back in to your chest using your "T" shape, before lowering your weights back down to your sides.**

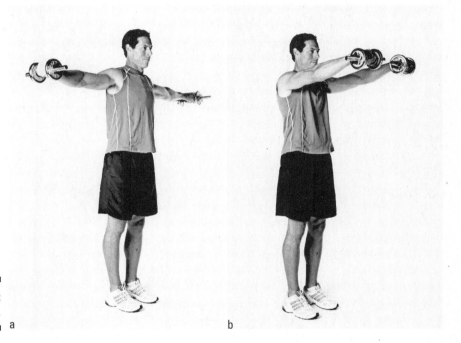

Figure 10-5:
T-raises.

a   b

While doing this exercise, remember these important tips:

✔ Keep your back straight during this exercise.

✔ Exhale as you lift the weights through your core to chest level and exhale as you lower back down to starting position.

Squat to overhead press

Combining two powerful movements or compound exercises is the way to go to strengthen your core with weights. This is a good overall upper and lower body exercise combining the squat and the overhead press.

To do this exercise, follow these steps:

1. **Starting with feet hip width apart and holding your dumbbells, bend your knees and squat down as if you were going to sit in a chair until your thighs are parallel with the floor (see Figure 10-6a).**

2. **Holding your weights in your hands at head level and even with your shoulders, press your weights upward until your elbows are straightened but not locked at the top of the movement (see Figure 10-6b).**

3. **Release your arms back down to shoulder level as you stand back up straight to starting position.**

4. **Repeat the movement in unison ten more times.**

Try to do the squat press movement slow and controlled to increase the tightening of your core muscles.

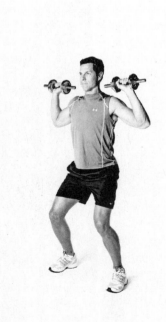 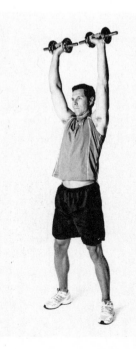

Figure 10-6:
Squat to overhead press.

a   b

Remember these tips while doing this exercise:

✔ Press your weights straight upwards during this exercise.

✔ Keep your back straight and stand tall. Don't lean forward.

Reverse lunges with weights

This reverse lunge with an added leg lift is done while you are holding weights. It's a great butt and back strengthener along with giving you killer abs from the extra knee lift.

To do this exercise, follow these steps:

1. **Holding your weights at waist level with palms facing each other, stand with your feet shoulder width apart. Step or lunge back with your right leg bending your left knee at a 90-degree angle (as shown in Figure 10-7a).**

2. **Holding your weights tightly at your waist, push through and straight up with your right knee as you contract your butt muscles on the left side of your body (see Figure 10-7b).**

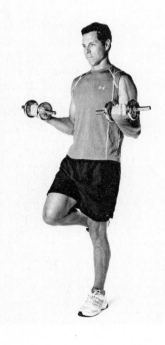
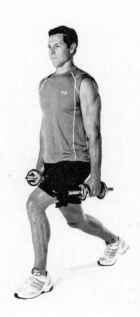

Figure 10-7:
Reverse lunges with weights.

a

b

3. **Hold the knee raise for a few seconds before returning your leg behind you to starting position.**

Maintain proper form by following these tips:

- ✔ Keep a straight back and not an arched one.
- ✔ Make sure you hold for a few seconds as you raise your knee.
- ✔ Pull your abs in tight and contract your butt muscles before doing this exercise.

Ab Central Machines

Ever go into the gym and see lots of ways to do a crunch except the old-fashioned way — on the floor? Ab machines are popular and are mostly made to stave off boredom because let's face it, doing crunches can get a little boring and a little difficult! Read on to find other ways to work your core that may add a little spice to your regular routine!

Ab roller

Looks like something that should be part of a jungle gym or at the very least something your kids might enjoy playing with, the ab roller is the half-dome-looking piece of equipment that you lie under on your back as you put your head on a little foam cushion for support. The movement is you rock forward as it helps you lift your shoulders off the ground, and it guides your spine through the natural curved movement when lifting. Definitely for beginners as it helps you take baby steps to getting an actual core workout or completing an abdominal crunch!

Ab board

With an ab board, it feels like your head is going to touch the ground because you are lying on your back with your legs above your hips and head as you tuck your feet under a roller. Great for sit-ups, crunches, and all abdominal exercises, the ab board provides you with a killer core workout and is a good piece of equipment to use if you already have a lot of core strength.

Because you are not just lying on your back on a flat surface but are at a 45-degree angle on an ab board, you are increasing the range of motion that you use to perform sit-ups, increasing the intensity of the exercise.

Ab wheel . . . yikes!

Inexpensive, yes. Convenient, oh yes. Easy to use? Forget it! The ab wheel really requires core strength along with balance and control to be able to use it. Picture this, starting with the wheel at your feet and your legs straight but hips up in the air (think downward dog in yoga), roll the wheel out until you are in pushup position. May sound easy but you have to control the movement or the wheel will take right off from under you and you'll be needing a new nose when it hits the floor. You can also use the ab wheel from a kneeling position instead of from a standing position but it is still a very advanced move. Again, the key word here is control and not many of us have what it takes to train with an ab wheel. Definitely something to work up to slowly.

Why build muscle to burn fat?

Using different forms of resistance, such as free weights and barbells, to reduce overall body fat by building muscle is the hottest and latest trend. Usually weights are incorporated as part of a circuit training program or added to some form of cardio training to be most effective. Using weights can help tone, add definition, and help reshape your body faster than any other form of exercise alone.

Here are a few of the many benefits you get from building muscle with resistance training:

- You burn 30 to 50 calories more per day at rest for each pound of muscle you put on. Imagine what that can do for you if you're active.

- Building bigger muscles boosts your metabolic rate (the rate at which you burn calories) and reduces overall body fat.

- Lean body mass burns more calories than fat does. So if you have more muscle, you can burn more calories while you sleep.

- It improves your posture as a result of strengthening and enhancing your back muscles, which help develop a strong spine.

- It increases your strength and muscle mass, which reduces the risk of osteoporosis due to the increase in bone density through weight training.

- It protects your joints and muscles from deterioration.

- It strengthens the connective tissue within your body

To burn the most amount of calories in the shortest amount of time, you need to work the larger muscle groups in your body. Next time you're doing a workout, try a few of these compound exercises rather than exercises that target individual muscles (as seen in this chapter):

- Squats

- Lat pulls

- Chest presses

These exercises are great examples of ways to burn the most calories in the shortest amount of time.

Part IV
Adding Variety to Your Core Routine

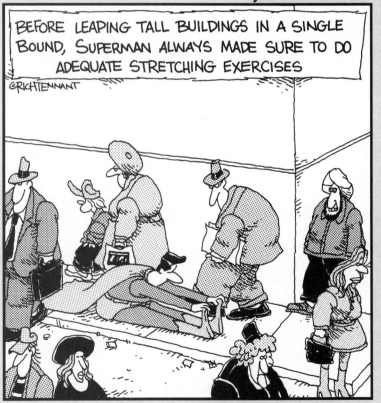

The 5th Wave   By Rich Tennant

BEFORE LEAPING TALL BUILDINGS IN A SINGLE BOUND, SUPERMAN ALWAYS MADE SURE TO DO ADEQUATE STRETCHING EXERCISES

In this part . . .

You will discover that no matter what principle of training you use, every technique uses core exercises to strengthen the body. Chapter 11 focuses on Pilates and the various exercises developed by Joseph Pilates himself that use core strength. Chapter 12 contains some of my favorite yoga exercises that you can do to develop a strong core with yoga poses — and help you relax a little bit and breathe a little slower.

Chapter 13 shows you how to use your own body weight as resistance for training and strengthening your core, like when you do a push-up or a triceps dip. It also shows you how to train with weights for your arms, back, butt, and legs as you carry your core along with you throughout the exercises.

Finally, Chapter 14 introduces a stretching routine designed to help you strengthen and stretch your core at the same time. I also address flexibility issues and the importance of stretchiness as you learn some fantastic stretches you can do to lengthen and lean out your midsection.

Chapter 11

Pilates Core Program

In This Chapter

▶ Practicing Pilates' principles

▶ Knowing why Pilates is a powerful core strengthener

▶ Getting ready for your Pilates core workout

▶ Combining diaphragmatic breathing with core exercises

*O*ne of the best fitness techniques that you can use on your body is Pilates. In fact, adapting the Pilates method for core training is a must as all Pilates movements that I know of originate in your core. There are so many ways that Pilates and core training go hand in hand to help strengthen the core. Check out a few of the examples below of how the exercises in this chapter are enhanced by using the Pilates method:

✔ Pilates encourages working the core by using the entire torso of the body in all of its exercises.

✔ Pilates is based in physiology and was created for reforming injuries by increasing core strength where all movements come from.

✔ Pilates uses the deep stabilizing muscles of your body to achieve balance and posture.

In this chapter, I give you some killer core exercise that will challenge you physically and even encourage you to breathe the Pilates way.

Getting Primed on the Principles of Pilates

Pilates is a mind *and* body experience. It's not just a way to get in shape or reform injuries; it also creates a real awareness of how your body works and where all your movements originate. The mindset you have when practicing Pilates is similar to the mindset of someone who's practicing martial arts. First, you must grasp the pebble from my hand, grasshopper. What I mean is that, in martial arts, you must first have the knowledge of the how and why to defend yourself before you go out and apply it. In Pilates, you must first understand the principles, or what you're trying to accomplish, before you do the exercises.

The Pilates method, just like yoga (see Chapter 12), has some basic principles. Here are the eight principles written by Joseph Pilates, the creator of Pilates, to help you perform his exercises as they were intended:

- **Breathing:** The best way to remember this principle is to exhale with effort. Using deep, diaphragmatic breathing (or breathing into your ribcage) allows you to create the proper flow and precision of each movement.

- **Range of motion:** This principle is basically flexibility, or how tight or loose your muscles are. Your range of motion affects your ability to stretch and extend, which are important to the Pilates method. People who have a limited range of motion will grow and benefit greatly from practicing Pilates.

- **Centering:** For this principle, you pull in your stomach muscles and engage your core, working from your center for every movement. Centering is the basis for all Pilates work and for using the ball because the ball is an unstable base. Pulling your navel in toward your spine means "sucking it in."

- **Controlling:** In this principle, you control your body's movements — each and every one of them. You know where everything is at all times. Having control of your body's movements creates body awareness that can enhance everything you do in life, from carrying a baby to stepping up on a ladder.

- **Stability:** For this principle, you want to *stabilize* your movements, or keep one body part still while another one is working. Stabilizing your lower back and not lifting your hips while you're lifting your legs is a good example of stability.

- **Flowing:** For this principle, you move freely through the movements, going from one to the next. The Pilates method has a real "dance" feel to it; you move smoothly through each exercise and finish with control.

- **Precision:** For this principle, you want to know where all your movements are coming from at all times. Being precise in each movement and being able to place your body and each limb where you would like it to be and where you would like it to end. Everything counts in Pilates and, for that reason, it takes a lot of focus and control to master it.

- **Opposition:** This principle is best described as working parts of your body in opposition to each other. Pressing your shoulders down while raising your arms or opening up your chest while bending at your waist are good examples of working in opposition.

Hitting the mat first

The art of Pilates has spread to athletes of all kinds along with professional dancers and just about everybody in between. In fact, anyone who wants to create long, lean muscles and correct postural alignment problems is doing himself a great service practicing Pilates. You can perform these exercises on an exercise mat (hence, the term *mat classes*), and you can use the mat exercises on the reformer.

To truly discover the who, what, where, when, and why of proper placement, I recommend learning Pilates mat exercises first before adding any equipment.

Putting all these principles together goes something like this: Teach your body to *flow* through movements with *precision* and *control*, working your body parts in *opposition* as you *breathe* through your limited *range of motion* and *center* yourself as you *stabilize*.

Using Pilates for Core Training

You get the following amazing benefits when you combine the Pilates method with specific core training:

- ✔ You'll get challenging exercises that require small movements and strength.
- ✔ You'll learn how to do Pilates mat exercises that don't require you to use a Pilates machine known as a reformer.
- ✔ You'll develop good muscle tone for your entire body because you're recruiting major muscle groups, which provides overall toning.
- ✔ You'll improve your flexibility.
- ✔ You'll gain better posture and improve your balance by breathing and holding yourself steady with Pilates exercises.
- ✔ You strengthen your body's core and the deeper abdominal muscles with Pilates exercises that other pieces of fitness equipment can't reach.
- ✔ You can adapt it to your own level of fitness by keeping either your upper body or lower body on the floor until you're ready to engage both by using your core strength.
- ✔ You'll elevate your heart rate with Pilates exercise because they require great strength and stamina.

Combining the principles and benefits of these two powerhouse forms of exercise can greatly improve your body's health. As with anything that's paired as a team, the results can be twice as good and twice as rewarding!

Preparing for Core Training the Pilates Way

You need a few things before you can do the Pilates exercises in this chapter. In this section, you find a list of the items you need and what you can do to make your workout go more smoothly.

You also discover how to find the *neutral spine* position that you need to use for every Pilates exercise. Make sure you take the time to try this position before you begin your workout.

Getting the Pilates stuff you need

Make sure that you have the following equipment for your Pilates-based core exercises:

- ✔ **Exercise mat:** You need an exercise mat to do the Pilates exercises in this chapter. An exercise mat allows you to kneel or lie on the floor so you can do the exercises more comfortably. You can use a yoga mat or you can try a small slip-resistant rug.

- ✔ **Comfortable clothing that's somewhat fitted:** You don't want your clothing to be too loose because it can inhibit your movements. The same goes for long hair, so be sure to pull it back before you begin your workout.

  Wearing something that allows you to see your stomach or abdominal muscles while working out is also a good idea so you can see whether you're breathing properly and keeping your ribcage open.

- ✔ **Work-out space:** Make sure that you work out in a space that has enough room for you to move and swing your arms and legs freely. You'll be lying on the floor quite a bit so make sure its clean and free of debris!

- ✔ **Water:** Staying hydrated is vital to your workout. It helps you recharge and keeps you from building up lactic acid in your muscles. *Lactic acid* is what makes you sore at the end of an intense workout. Keep a water bottle handy so you can sip it throughout your exercise session — it'll provide you with better stamina so you can last longer.

- ✔ **Doctor's approval:** As with any new workout, consulting your physician before you begin a new workout is important. If at any time during this workout you feel any pain, stop what you're doing and rest quietly on your mat or stretch yourself out. A good rule when exercising is, "if in doubt, leave it out!"

✔ **Bare feet:** Leave your shoes and socks off for these exercises, but save them for when you're using weights or doing cardio exercises. Because you need to grip the floor with your feet, going barefoot for this workout is best.

Unveiling the path to a neutral spine

One of the principle factors in practicing Pilates is *neutral spine*. The ultimate goal in trying to achieve a neutral spine is to keep the natural curve of your spine without overcorrecting it.

In other words, you want to stabilize your back, your hipbones, and your pelvis so they're on the same plane.

To try neutral spine and to see whether you're maintaining that natural curve in your spine, do the following:

1. **Lie with your back and feet flat on the floor and your knees bent at a 90-degree angle.**

2. **Flatten your lower back by pressing it into the floor.**

   Now you can feel the difference between neutral spine and a flat back.

3. **Arch your back slightly by lifting your hips up.**

   Now you can feel the differences between an arched back, a flat back, and the natural curve in your spine (or neutral spine).

If you were standing, your pelvis would drop straight down. The proper way to describe a neutral spine while standing up would be neither arched nor tilted forward. Just as your car has a neutral position in which it doesn't move forward or backward, the same goes for a neutral spine.

Breathing the Pilates way

Breathing requires very specific attention in Pilates. Pilates demands deep diaphragmatic breathing done by expanding your ribcage (and belly) then letting it close as you exhale. Breathing by expansion of the ribcage is predominantly caused by the intercostals. The diaphragm basically depresses the floor of the thorax causing the belly to expand. By placing your hand on your belly, you can become more aware of the area you're using to breathe with the Pilates method. Below is a breathing exercise you can practice before beginning your workout so you can get the most out of doing the following exercises.

Use your hand to feel your abdomen and ribcage rise and fall.

To properly breathe the Pilates way, follow these steps:

1. **Lie on your back and bend your knees, keeping your feet flat on the floor.**

    Your legs should be hip-distance apart.

2. **Rest one hand on your belly and one hand on your ribcage.**

3. **Take a deep breath, allowing your ribcage and to rise as your belly fills with air.**

4. **Exhale, making sure that all the air leaves your belly and your ribcage moves back together.**

5. **Repeat immediately after your exhale.**

    Inhale to the count of ten and exhale to the count of ten for several breaths.

While you're doing your Pilates breathing:

- ✔ Keep your back pressed into the floor so you can feel your ribcage expand.
- ✔ Inhale through your nose.
- ✔ Keep your feet flat on the floor so you can see your ribcage expand on each inhale.

Trying Out Beginner Pilates Core Care

This series of exercises incorporates the breathing technique I show you in this chapter to help you create body awareness and get you through this workout. And of course, *breathing* is one of the eight Pilates principles.

The plank and the bridge are modified Pilates exercises that require *stamina* and *balance*. And even a few more of your Pilates principles, such as *centering* and *opposition,* appear here.

You should perform these exercises in the following order to allow your chest to open up before you release your back.

Pilates bridge

The Pilates bridge is a variation of the classic bridge position that Chapter 9 illustrates. This version is more difficult because you have to lift your hips higher while stabilizing your core.

You need to incorporate your core muscles (remember, from your ribcage to your hips) or stabilizers to help you maintain the strength in your lower back and lift in your hips throughout this exercise.

To do this exercise, follow these steps:

1. **Lie on your back with your knees bent and feet flat on the floor. Take a deep breath in as you squeeze your butt and lift your hips up off the floor (see Figure 11-1a).**

   Your arms will be straight and alongside your body.

2. **Exhale as you lift your hips high enough to make a straight line with your body from your shoulders to your knees. Make sure you can see the tops of your knees (as Figure 11-1b shows).**

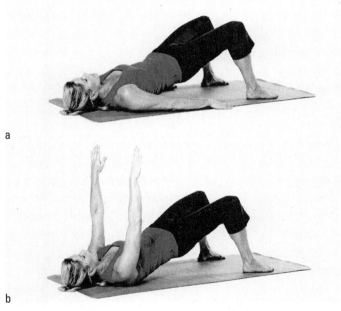

a

Figure 11-1:
Pilates
bridge.

b

   Be sure not to place any strain on your neck by lifting too high. Lift up only as high as hip level.

3. **Hold for a few seconds using the support of your arms and your breathing to help you maintain the position.**

4. **Exhale as you slowly roll your spine back down onto the floor one vertebra at a time.**

Complete five to ten repetitions, depending on your individual fitness level.

When doing the Pilates bridge, remember to:

- ✔ Inhale as you lift up your hips.

- ✔ Keep your eyes cast toward the ceiling to help you keep your neck straight during the lift.

- ✔ Remain relaxed and think of using your breath to help you through this exercise. Don't let your shoulders tense up.

The plank

The plank position works your core muscles while it also works your upper body. It strengthens and lengthens your body by activating your stabilizing muscles and this exercise is done just how it sounds: keeping your body straight in a plank position, just like a plank of wood.

To do this exercise, follow these steps:

1. **With your hands pressed down and your fingers facing forward, place your hands shoulder-width apart on the floor in front of you and your legs straight behind you (see Figure 11-2a).**

   Your arms will be straight underneath your shoulders.

2. **Exhale as you slowly lift your body off the floor, contracting your abdominals until your arms and elbows are straight (see Figure 11-2b).**

   You need to contract your chest muscles and engage your upper body for additional support.

3. **Hold this position for a few seconds before lowering your body slowly back down to the floor.**

   Complete five to ten repetitions, depending on your individual fitness level.

To get the most out of the plank, you need to:

- ✔ Press into the floor and squeeze you glutes while you're in the plank position.

- ✔ Keep your neck in line with your spine as you do when you're standing.

- ✔ Keep your back straight and long — don't let your back arch or sag.

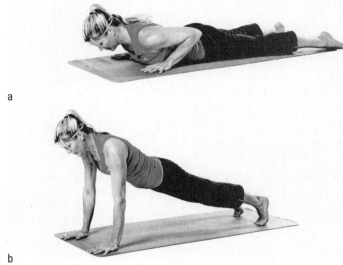

Figure 11-2:
Pilates
plank.

a

b

Roll downs

The roll down exercise is just as it sounds. Using a slow and controlled movement, you roll your torso and upper back down to the floor and then back up.
This exercise helps you develop strong abdominal and lower back muscles,
which help you maintain a strong and healthy core.

Using an exercise mat will make your back more comfortable during this
exercise.

To do this exercise, follow these steps:

1. **Sit up tall with your knees bent and feet flat on the floor. Imagine a string
   is lifting you up from the top of your head and is attached to the ceiling.**

2. **Pulling your belly button in toward your spine to activate your
   abdominal muscles, extend your arms straight out in front of you (as
   Figure 11-3a shows).**

3. **Slowly roll your spine down toward the floor one vertebra at a time,
   making a "C" shape with your lower back (see Figure 11-3b).**

4. **Roll all the way down until you are lying flat on the floor and your
   arms are at your sides.**

5. **Slowly roll yourself back up into starting position using your core muscles.**

   Complete five repetitions.

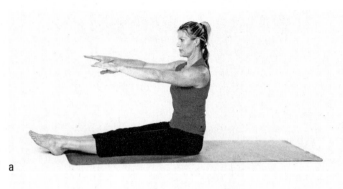

a

b

Get results with roll downs by remembering to:

- ✔ Use a slow and controlled movement when rolling your spine down to the floor.
- ✔ Use your breath to help you focus on holding your position.
- ✔ Keep your arms extended out in front of you as you roll down.

Swimming

This exercise trains your back and entire core to work together while at the same time strengthening your abdominals. Remember, keeping your back strong and flexible and your abdominals tight and strong is the best prevention against low back problems.

To do this exercise, follow these steps:

1. **Lie flat on your belly on a mat or the floor with your arms stretched out in front of you and your legs stretched out behind you (as shown in Figure 11-4a).**

2. **Pulling your belly button in, simultaneously lift your upper back and head off the floor along with your right arm and left leg.**

3. **Switch arms and legs and begin swimming as you alternate your arms and legs (see Figure 11-4b).**

   Imagine that strings are attached to your hand and foot and that the strings are gently pulling your arm and leg away from each other, not up. You want to get the lengthening in your abdominal muscles and your spine, not shortening or compressing it.

4. **Squeeze your butt muscles and swim continuously for 24 strokes or beats.**

   Lower your arms and legs and return to the floor.

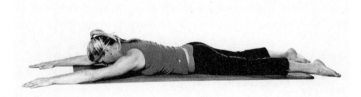

a

Figure 11-4:
Lifting your opposite arm and leg in the Superman pose.

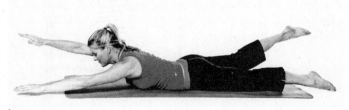

b

While doing this exercise:

- ✔ Keep your abdominals tight. Lax abdominals may place undue stress on your lower back muscles.

- ✔ Avoid arching your back.

- ✔ Make sure that you don't lift your pubic bone up off the mat.

The hundred

One of the most common Pilates exercises, the hundred is a real core strengthener. Because you're lifting your head and shoulders off the floor as you squeeze your inner thighs together, you're engaging both the upper and lower abdominal core area. Great exercise!

To do this exercise, follow these steps:

1. **Lie on your back with your knees up in the air forming a 90-degree angle with your hips.** Squeeze your inner thighs together in a "tabletop" position.

2. **Maintaining neutral spine, place your arms straight alongside your body and just off the floor with palms facing down (see Figure 11-5a).**

3. **Lift your head and shoulder blades until they are just off the mat.**

4. **Inhale slowly and pulse your arms just above floor level for five beats then exhale slowly and pulse your arms for five beats, making up ten beats all together (see Figure 11-5b).**

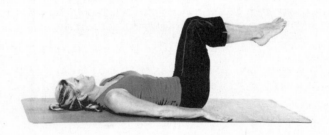

a

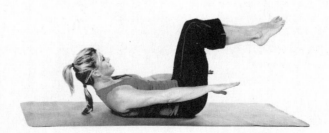

Figure 11-5:
The
hundred.

b

Slowly roll back down to the mat and repeat ten times to make a total of a "hundred" beats.

Here's what you can't forget about the hundred:

✔ Use your abs to hold you up and not your neck to avoid straining your neck muscles.

✔ Put one hand behind your neck halfway through this exercise at 50 beats if the strain on your neck becomes too much.

✔ Keep your shoulder blades back and down — don't let them rise up.

Single-leg stretch

The single-leg stretch is a wonderful core Pilates exercise to teach you how to stabilize your spine while working your abs and back. It's almost like doing a bicycle crunch except it's done more slowly and it calls upon your core strength to pull each knee in toward you and hold.

To do this exercise, follow these steps:

1. **Sit up tall on the floor with your feet flat and knees bent. Slowly roll down as you pull one knee into your chest and straighten the other leg out at a 45-degree angle to the floor (as shown is Figure 11-6a).**

   Your shoulder blades will remain off the floor to engage your core.

2. **Hold your bent knee gently with both hands and switch legs two times on one inhale and two times on one exhale (see Figure 11-6b).**

   Repeat for eight total breaths in all.

When you do the single leg stretch:

✔ Lift your head high enough to engage your abs and not strain your neck.

✔ Keep your belly button pulled into your spine as you exhale.

✔ Inhale for two beats and exhale for two beats emphasizing proper Pilates breathing.

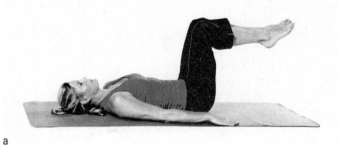

a

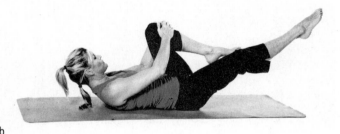

Figure 11-6:
Single-leg
stretch.

b

Rising swan

This exercise strengthens your back and butt along with stretching out your abdominals. I love to do this exercise as part of my cooldown and finish by pressing back on my heels and resting my upper body on them for support in child's pose or resting position.

To do this exercise, follow these steps:

1. **Lie down on your belly with your forearms on the mat supporting your upper back. Keep your arms at your sides in a sphinx pose (as shown in Figure 11-7a).**

2. **Slowly rise up higher with your upper back, gently lifting your head and straightening your arms by pressing your hands into the mat (see Figure 11-7b).**

3. **Hold this position for a few seconds before lowering back down to the floor.**

Rise to the challenge by making sure that you:

✔ Pull your belly button in and squeeze your butt muscles.

✔ Lift only as high as is comfortable to you to avoid placing any undo stress on your lower back — don't lift too high.

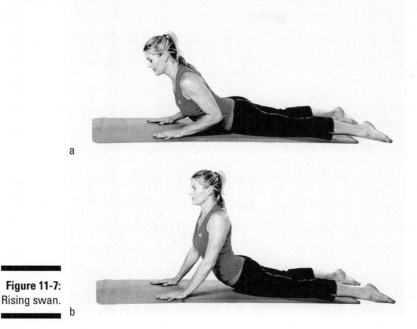

a

b

Figure 11-7:
Rising swan.

Side kicks

This exercises targets the core by using a movement that comes directly from the abdominals and back. It also helps you with stability, as you have to keep your body steady as you move your legs freely.

To do this exercise, follow these steps:

1. **Lie on your side with your legs stretched out and a little bit in front of your body (see Figure 11-8a).**

2. **Prop your head up on your elbow and place your front arm palm down on the floor in front of you.**

3. **Flex your foot as you kick your top leg out in front of you pulsing it once before switching directions and swinging it behind you (see Figure 11-8b).**

4. **Complete ten repetitions on each side.**

Keep these tips in mind while doing side kicks:

✔ Press your weight into the front of your palm to help keep your torso steady and maintain balance.

✔ Keep your neck relaxed and long.

  ▮ ✔ Avoid letting your upper body move as you swing your leg.

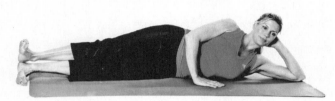

a

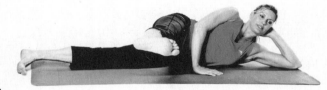

Figure 11-8:
Side kicks.

b

What is the Pilates method?

Joseph Pilates, creator of the Pilates method, was born in 1881 and died in 1967. He was an accomplished circus performer, gymnast, and a notable boxer. Having many injuries from all the activities that he had participated in, Joseph Pilates came up with a series of exercises to overcome them. After perfecting these exercises that worked for him in rehabilitating his injuries, he wanted to pass this series of exercises onto ailing patients so they could recover, too, so he made crude pieces of equipment out of springs and pulleys to use with hospital beds. The result was that patients could get physical rehabilitation and work out while lying in bed. Genius!

Fast-forward many years later when Joseph Pilates turned these crude machines into what's now known as the Pilates *reformer,* or the Pilates *bed,* which can be used with more than 100 exercises devised by Joseph Pilates known as the *Pilates method.* The fact that the Pilates method today actually grew out of its roots and remained true to what it was created for is amazing. And, boy, is it ever still around today!

Chapter 12

Yoga Core

In recent years, yoga has become mainstream and is now practiced by yogis, weekend warriors, and you guessed it — even regular folks! And that is because people have discovered that yoga is a real workout — not just a few simple stretches or strength poses . . . no, it actually is a workout that will kick your butt!

In this chapter, I demonstrate some classic yoga poses that will prepare your core for any yoga class you walk into. As the following yoga poses demonstrate, you have to possess great core strength along with a strong upper body to maintain the following exercises (or as they're called in yoga, "poses"). The downward dog and the sun salutation, both shown in this chapter, are just a few examples of poses that will challenge your body and your mind.

Doing yoga poses is very challenging so you're not alone if you want to rest in some of the poses, and that's what child's pose is for. So relax when you need to during the following workouts, and take your time stretching back in child's pose to take a break when you need to.

Benefits of Doing Yoga

It's true, you'll need to be flexible to practice yoga but it's a bit of a catch-22. Yoga can give you the strength that you need to be flexible, but because everybody's range of motion differs due to different degrees of elasticity in each individual's joints, some people will be able to stretch like a rubber band, whereas others might have a hard time touching their toes (that's right men, I'm talking to you!).

The goal of all these yoga poses is to help extend your range of motion, which helps strengthen your core so that all the activities you do throughout the day become easier and maybe even — dare I say — effortless.

So whatever group you fall into, the flexible group or the inflexible group (men), here is a list of benefits you'll get from doing yoga and how yoga can help build strength and flexibility:

- Yoga helps relieve lower back pain by elongating the key muscles that control the pelvic and back area, such as the hamstrings, lumbar muscles, hip flexors, and glutes.

- Yoga poses heat up the core muscles of your body, which makes performing all movements easier throughout the day.

- Yoga helps you expend less energy during the day because of increased flexibility, which results in all your movements being made easier.

- Yoga reduces stress by increasing the blood supply to tight, tense muscles.

- Yoga gives you better posture by realigning and strengthening the muscles that support coordination and movement.

- Yoga reduces injuries by helping you gain better control over your body's movements.

You can do the yoga poses in this chapter before you begin your day or even before you begin your regular workout. They will not only get your circulation going, but also will help you gain some strength and inner peace before you begin your day.

Taking It Slowly and Breathing

Breathing is one of the fundamental principles of practicing yoga. And it's also one of the fundamental principles in life — we all need to breathe! Once you understand that the breath you take is literally your neighbor's — (in some shape or form) then you can begin to understand the mindset of yoga practitioners . . . everyone is connected through their breath.

It's true, breathing through a yoga pose helps you through the exercise but it also connects everyone to each other as they breathe the same air and exchange atoms floating through the air. Breathing takes on a much bigger meaning in yoga because it becomes a life force, or something you need to exist and connect you to all of humanity and the world around us.

As you do the poses in this chapter, breathe in slowly through your nose as you feel the air hit the back of your throat. As you exhale, let the breath out through your mouth and release all the tension from the pose to help clear your mind for the next one.

Flowing through your core movements

When you bend your body in different ways, you gain the ability to work entirely different muscle groups. When you stretch muscles in opposition, you strengthen them and improve flexibility at the same time. The technical terms for all the bending you'll be doing are flexion, extension, abduction, and adduction.

The following is a short explanation of what it's called when you're bending every which way in yoga:

✔ *Flexion* is bending, or decreasing the angle, at the joint. Flexing your knee toward your butt is a good example of knee flexion.

✔ *Extension* means straightening, or increasing the angle, at the joint as you would do when you are straightening your knee.

✔ *Abduction* and *adduction* also work in opposition to each other and are terms best described as working your arms or legs toward the body or away from it. If you bring your legs or arms toward the center line of your body you're adducting them. If you take your arms and move them away from the center of your body, you're abducting them.

Whichever way you happen to be bending, using slow, controlled movements gives you the best results and helps you achieve strength and flexibility at the same time.

To test this theory, try holding your breath during one of the yoga poses in this chapter and see how difficult it is to do (but not too long or you'll pass out!). Breathing is a life force, and in yoga it's used to enhance your workout and increase your flexibility. So just breathe!

Strong Core Poses

In the following yoga poses, I suggest taking it easy and working up slowly. I always suggest trying each pose lightly first before trying to fully execute it to its fullest capacity. Never push or strain, especially in yoga, because it's not about competing or pushing yourself to the limit; instead, yoga is about feeling the movement and energy in your core and throughout your body so you can stay in touch with what body part you're actually working.

Feel free to mix and match the following poses any way you like. However, in yoga they do follow a specific order and I've written them that way here in this chapter. I find that doing them in the following order works best because you get your blood flowing first before you jump into a full-body workout.

For the following yoga sequence, use an exercise mat or yoga mat to help you grip the floor with your toes and cushion your knees for comfort.

Downward dog

Ever watch your dog wake up and stretch his body out with his paws extended in front of him with his butt in the air? You guessed it, that's where the name of this pose comes from. The downward-facing dog energizes your entire body because your head is lower than your heart, fueling fresh blood to your brain. It also works the entire back by stretching out your spine and requires great ab and hip strength to support the movement.

To do this pose, follow these easy steps:

1. **Start on your hands and knees, making sure your hands are directly beneath your shoulders and your knees are directly under your hips.**

   Spread your palms out wide on the floor.

2. **Exhale as you lift and straighten your arms and raise your hips up behind you and toward the ceiling. Straighten your legs but don't lock your knees as you let your head fall down between your arms, lining up your ears with your arms (shown in Figure 12-1).**

3. **Breathe as you press your heels toward the floor and your head toward your feet.**

   Hold the movement for a few seconds before you release back down to your hands and knees.

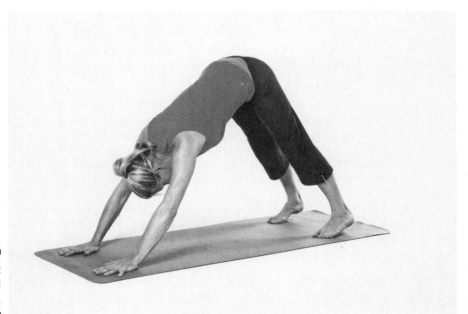

Figure 12-1:
Downward
dog.

While doing this pose, remember to:

✔ Allow your head and neck to relax toward the floor by casting your eyes downward.

✔ Exhale with effort as you relax your body and stretch toward the floor.

✔ Press your heels as far as you can toward the floor. Don't let your heels come off the floor.

Plank

The plank position works your core muscles while it also works your upper body. It strengthens and lengthens your body by activating your stabilizing muscles.

In yoga, the plank is done as part of a series of poses called the sun salutation, which I cover in the following exercises. Keeping your body straight in a plank position — just like a plank of wood — is the perfect core pose for any yoga practice.

To do this pose, follow these steps:

1. **With your hands pressed down and your fingers facing forward, place your hands shoulder-width apart on the floor in front of you and your legs straight behind you (as Figure 12-2a shows).**

   Your arms will be straight underneath your shoulders.

2. **Exhale as you slowly lift your body off the floor, contracting your abdominals until your arms and elbows are straight (see Figure 12-2b).**

   Breathe as you contract your abdominal muscles and engage your upper body for additional support.

3. **Hold this position for a few seconds before lowering your body slowly back down to the floor.**

   Complete five to ten times, depending on your individual fitness level.

While practicing the plank, be sure to:

✔ Press into the floor and squeeze your glutes while you're in the plank position.

✔ Keep your neck in line with your spine as you do when you're standing.

✔ Keep your back straight and long. *Don't* let your back arch or sag to the floor.

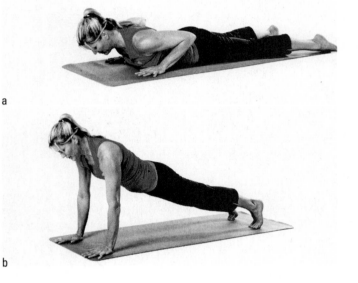

a

b

Figure 12-2:
Your hands
should be
on the floor
and in line
with your
shoulders.

Cobra

The abs, back, and shoulders are targeted in the cobra pose. The cobra pose also stimulates the internal organs like the kidneys and liver in your lower back area to help them function better.

To do this pose, follow these steps:

1. **Lie on the floor with your stomach down as you place your forearms flat on the floor. Let your forehead rest on the floor also.**

2. **Inhale as you tighten your back and abdominal muscles pressing your forearms against the floor to raise your chest and head (Figure 12-3).**

3. **Exhale as you release your torso and head slowly back down to the floor to starting position.**

Complete three times, remembering to breathe deeply each time.

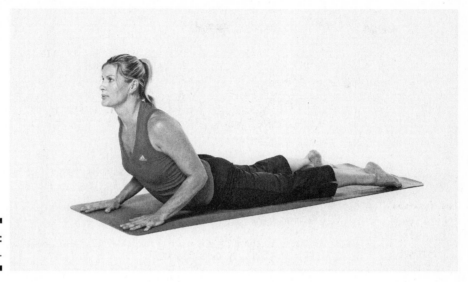

Figure 12-3:
Cobra pose.

You get the best results if you:

- ✔ Use a yoga mat or a towel support for your head to rest on.
- ✔ Exhale before you extend your forearms and tighten your core muscles.
- ✔ Press the tops of your feet into the floor during this pose.

Stretchy and Sticky Core Poses

Breathing, relaxing, and concentration are what the next four yoga poses are all about. The cat/cow is done in another chapter (see Chapter 15) and is used as a yoga pose to release the back. The forward bend also is used to release and stretch the back and lower body as it extends toward the floor. The child's pose is known as the relaxing pose and is used resting your body as a baby or child would do to rest. It is used throughout a yoga class to rest your body and help prepare it for the next exercise. The corpse pose is done just like it sounds, and is always the final relaxation pose done in any yoga class. These are done in a specific sequence according to classic yoga poses but you can do them in any order you like.

Cat/Cow

Not only does this pose help make your back feel better, but also the cat/cow improves the range of motion in your spine, enhances strength and coordination of the muscles around your spine, and improves core muscle awareness in your entire back — all factors that make your lower back feel better and stay healthy.

To do this pose, follow these steps:

1. **Get on the floor on your hands and knees with your hands directly under your shoulders and your knees directly under your hips.**

2. **Inhale and arch your back, lifting your tailbone and eyes toward the ceiling (see Figure 12-4a).**

3. **Hold the stretch for a few seconds then release the position back to neutral spine, and inhale again.**

4. **Exhale and contract your abdominals, rounding your back like an angry cat (see Figure 12-4b).**

5. **Hold this position for a few seconds and then release back to neutral spine.**

   Repeat this pose four to six times.

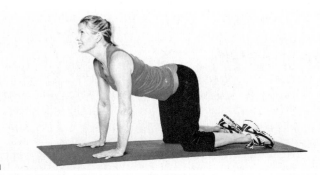

a

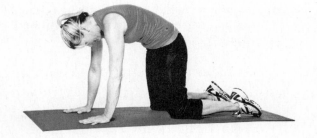

Figure 12-4:
Cat/Cow
pose.

b

While doing the cat/cow pose:

- ✔ Pull your belly button toward your spine.
- ✔ Keep the movement in your pelvis and lower back, not in your shoulders.
- ✔ Avoid tensing up your shoulders and neck.
- ✔ Remember not to overextend your neck while doing the old cow position.

Forward bend

 If you have lower back problems, the forward bend may not be right for you. You can do a forward bend from a lying position, sitting position, or from a standing position like I use here. It is similar to touching your toes; however, the difference is you will be resting in this pose as you place your palms on the floor . . . or try to anyway!

This pose stretches out your back, butt, and hamstrings as you bring your upper body to the floor.

To do this pose, follow these steps:

1. **With your feet wider than shoulder-width apart, inhale as you extend your arms over head.**

2. **Lean forward from your hips with your chest toward the floor. Keep your back straight the entire time (see Figure 12-5).**

3. **Place your hands or palms on the floor on front of you. If you feel a strain in the back of your legs, soften your knees and rest your hands on your shins.**

   Place your hands on the floor in front of you, if you feel you need an additional stretch.

4. **After holding the stretch for a few seconds, roll your body back up into starting position.**

   Complete three to five times as you breathe into the pose.

When you do the forward bend, remember to:

- ✔ Hold your stretch before slowly rolling back up into starting position.
- ✔ Widen your feet to get closer to the floor to intensify this stretch.
- ✔ Keep your back straight and bend from your waist. Don't arch your back at all.

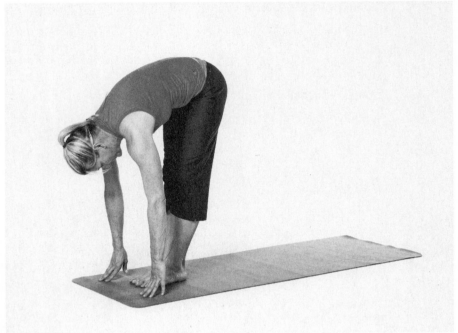

Figure 12-5:
Forward
bend.

Child's pose

Ah, my favorite yoga pose! Ha! I referred to it before as the resting pose and that's just what it is: a short rest in between or just before the most difficult poses begin.

The child's pose helps elongate and stretch your *quadriceps* (the muscles that run along the *front* of your upper leg) as you rest your body weight on your legs. Most people who have tight quads usually also have tight *hamstrings* (the muscles that run along the *back* of the upper legs) so this is a great pose for both areas.

You can rest in child's pose with your arms extended or outreached on the floor in front of you to get an extra shoulder stretch. Or just keep them at your sides to rest and relax.

To do this pose, follow these steps:

1. **Kneel on the floor with your knees about hip width apart. As you exhale, sit back on your heels, resting your torso on your thighs (as shown in Figure 12-6).**

2. **Lay your arms back on the floor behind you beside your torso.**

3. **Breathe and close your eyes, relaxing into the pose for five breaths.**

4. **Slowly return back to kneeling position, letting your blood and breath return to your body before standing.**

   Repeat five times.

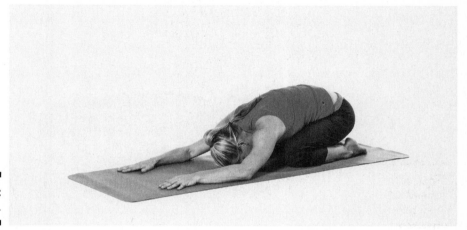

Figure 12-6:
Child's pose.

Make the best of your inner child through pose, by remember to:

✔ Keep your arms alongside your body for extra relaxation.

✔ Keep your eyes closed as you relax into the pose.

✔ Keep your head straight with your forehead on the floor. Don't turn your head to either side.

Corpse pose

And last but not least is the final resting pose known as the corpse pose. Always done as the final pose in any yoga class, this classic pose helps you get in touch with your breathing and focus on relaxing your body.

To do this exercise, follow these simple steps:

1. **Lie on your back on a yoga mat or towel with your arms resting alongside your body and your palms facing down (see Figure 12-7).**

2. **As you inhale, slowly raise your arms above your head for a more active pose. Otherwise, keep your arms alongside your body and breathe long inhales through your nose and exhale through your mouth.**

3. **Lie in corpse pose breathing deeply for three to five minutes or for six to eight deep yoga breaths.**

4. **Hold this stretch for a few seconds before you release your arm. Repeat on your other side.**

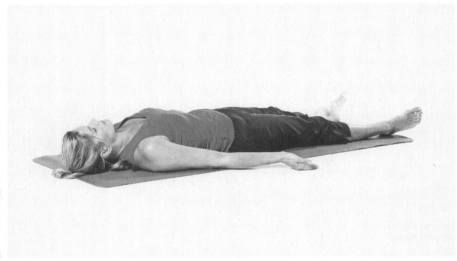

Figure 12-7:
Corpse
pose.

Taking In My Favorite Abs Tightener: Sun Salutation

The next series of poses puts together many of the different poses discussed earlier in this chapter as a final test so to speak Not to worry — it's not a test, but it is a nice combination of the plank, cobra, forward bend, and child's pose that you've come to love. So have fun putting all these moves together!

Make all your movements flow one right into the other, as you breathe and focus on your breath.

The sun salutation is a series of movements combined to help you wake up your body and get your blood flowing. It's great to do first thing in the morning or last thing before you go to bed.

To flow through this sequence of poses known as sun salutation, follow these poses in order.

Standing position

Start in standing position with your feet hip width apart. Place your palms in front of your chest in prayer position (see Figure 12-8).

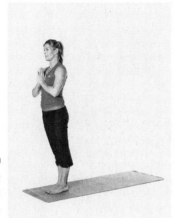

Figure 12-8:
Standing
position.

Arms raised overhead

Inhale and raise your arms overhead with your palms still together (see Figure 12-9). Arch your back as you look up toward the ceiling.

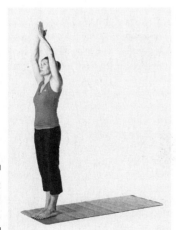

Figure 12-9:
Arms raised
overhead.

Forward bend

Exhale as you bend forward from your hips. Place your hands on the floor in front of you as you soften your knees (see Figure 12-10).

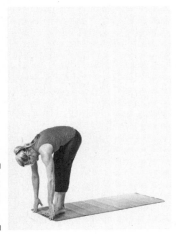

Figure 12-10:
Forward
bend.

Step back lunge position

Inhale as you bend your left knee and step your right foot back into a lunge position (see Figure 12-11).

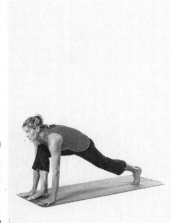

Figure 12-11:
Step back
lunge
position.

Plank position

Exhale as you step your left foot back beside your right and hold a plank or push-up position (see Figure 12-12).

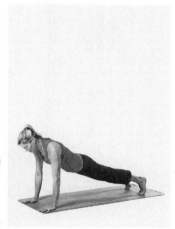

Figure 12-12:
Plank
position.

Inchworm

Inhale and exhale as you lower your knees from push up position and push your chin and chest to the floor. Keep your butt in the air and move like an inchworm (as seen in Figure 12-13).

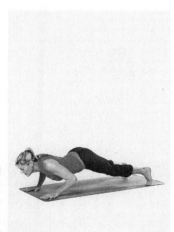

Figure 12-13:
Inchworm
pose.

Cobra position

Inhale as you slide your chest along the floor and arch back into cobra position (see Figure 12-14).

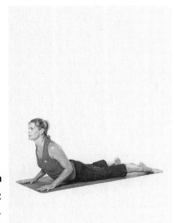

Figure 12-14:
Cobra.

Downward dog

Exhale as you turn your toes under and raise your hips up toward the ceiling. Keep both hands on the floor as you bring your chest toward your knees in downward dog position (see Figure 12-15).

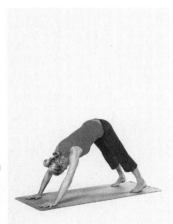

Figure 12-15:
Downward dog.

Lunge position

You are now returning to lunge position by stepping your right foot forward between your hands and looking straight ahead (see Figure 12-16).

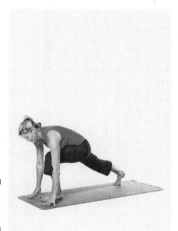

Figure 12-16:
Lunge pose.

Forward bend

Exhale as you step your left foot forward to meet your right foot. Soften you knees as you fold into forward bend (see Figure 12-17).

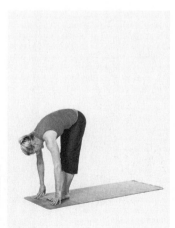

Figure 12-17:
Forward
bend.

Arms raised overhead

Inhale as you reach your arms out to the sides of your body in an airplane position and return them up above your head (see Figure 12-18).

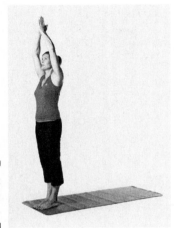

Figure 12-18:
Arms raised
overhead.

Prayer position

Exhale as you return your hands into prayer position in front of your chest (see Figure 12-19).

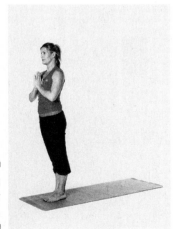

Figure 12-19:
Prayer
position.

Repeat the sequence six times leading with your right foot the first time and alternating with your left foot for an equal amount of times.

Putting the poses together

After you become more proficient at doing each pose of the sun salutation, use Figure 12-20 to see the entire sequence so that you can perform the sun salutation more fluidly. Do the poses in this order: (a) standing position, (b) arms raised overhead, (c) forward bend, (d) step back lunge position, (e) plank position, (f) inchworm, (g) cobra, (h) downward dog, (i) lunge position, (j) forward bend, (k) arms raised overhead, and (l) prayer position.

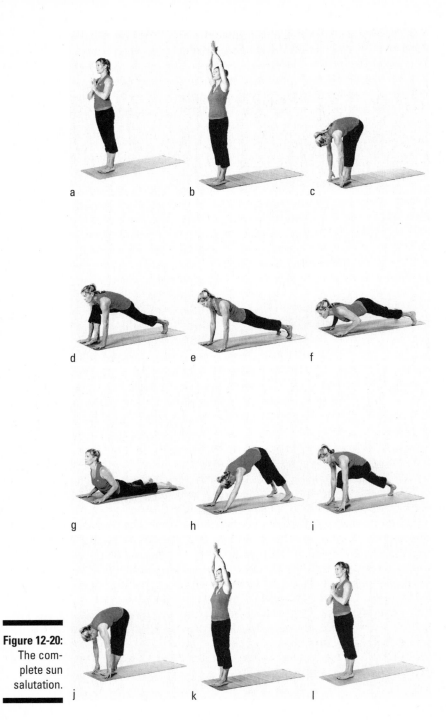

Figure 12-20:
The complete sun salutation.

Chapter 13

Working Your Core While Exercising Other Muscles

In This Chapter

▶ Building a stronger core with the help of your upper body

▶ Strengthening the core as you recruit your lower body

▶ Performing interval training with the assistance of your core

▶ Using the resistance of your own body weight to build your core

Core training doesn't result in great, sculpted abs alone. Because your core consists of all the musculature, front and back, starting at your knees and going all the way up to your chest, your core actually includes several large muscle groups. All these muscles must work together to execute all movements your body makes. If your core is weak, your movements will be weak, and you won't be able execute in the gym or in everyday life. When you work your arms and legs and other body parts, you transition all those movements through your core. So while you're busy toning those other body parts, you're also toning your core.

Because muscle tone is a good indicator of overall fitness, the best way to tell whether people are in shape is to look at their arms and legs as well as their midsection. For women and men, maintaining muscle in the arms can be difficult because they lose muscle tone as they age. Even with all the lifting, pulling, and picking up you do throughout the day, you need to work your arms and legs to keep them beautifully toned in addition to keeping your body fat low to see your muscles.

In this chapter, I incorporate many different muscle groups in the core exercises so you're working more than just your core. The exercises contribute to a well-balanced workout that will keep you looking fit and give with a sleek upper and lower body.

Visualizing Working Muscles

I always like to know which muscle I'm working during a workout so I can visualize it getting bigger and stronger. Thinking about the body part that you're exercising helps you concentrate and focus, for better results. Because your body is made up of many different muscles, here's a brief overview of the muscles you use in the workouts in this chapter.

Targeted upper-body muscles

Here's an overview of the upper-body muscles you'll be using in the following exercises:

- **Biceps muscles:** The *biceps* start at the top of the shoulder joint and run down into the forearm. When you use a pulling motion with any exercise, you recruit the biceps. The biceps muscles are primarily responsible for bending your arms.

- **Triceps muscles:** The *triceps* are a little more complicated. They consist of three different muscles that run along the backs of your arms. The triceps are responsible for straightening your elbows. Anytime you press something down or are pushing something away from you (whether it be pushing in front or pushing overhead), you use the triceps.

- **Forearm muscles:** The *forearms,* or lower arms, run from your elbow down to your wrist. These muscles often get neglected because many people know that the forearms get some exercise by working the biceps and triceps.

- **Shoulder muscles:** Finally, the *shoulder muscles* tie all these muscles together, so to speak. The shoulder muscle consists of three muscles, known as the *anterior, medial,* and *posterior deltoids;* together these muscles are called the *deltoids,* or just the "delts." The delts help rotate your arm and raise it up and down and front to back. Anytime you raise your arms over your head, you work or use your shoulder muscles.

Targeted lower-body muscles

Here's an overview of the lower-body muscles you'll be using in the following exercises:

✔ **Hamstrings:** Located on the back of your upper leg (just under your butt) and behind your knee are the hamstrings. Many people have tight hamstrings from sitting at their desk all day and can alleviate the tightness with proper stretching and exercises that strengthen this large muscle group. Lunges are a good exercise that is found in this chapter to help strengthen your hamstrings along with your core.

✔ **Quadriceps:** The group of four muscles that are located in the front of the upper leg are known as the quadriceps or quads. They are all used in movements that concern the knee joint like running, squatting, jumping, and walking.

✔ **Glutes:** The glutes are made up of three muscles but (no pun intended) the largest of the three muscles is the gluteus maximus better known as the butt! The gluteus maximus is what gives the appearance or actual shape to your backside.

Refresher for Using Proper Form with Weights

I discuss using weights to build a stronger core in Chapter 4. I am also including a brief refresher in this chapter on that information…just in case you don't feel like flipping!

When you use weights, you get better results — but you have to use weights without hurting yourself. The following list rounds up some tips to avoid injury:

✔ **Keep your shoulders back and down.** If your shoulders tense up and float up around your ears, you're using too much weight. Not good! Keep your shoulders pressed down and back, for good posture and to avoid injury.

✔ **Keep your chest lifted.** Keep your chest or sternum up and lifted so you don't hunch over and hurt your lower back. You need to use your core muscles to keep your chest up, so you work on both body parts and posture at once.

✔ **Keep wrists in line with elbows.** To keep you from hurting your joints and pulling a muscle, never bend your wrists when lifting weights. Keep them on the same plane with your elbows.

✔ **Keep your hips in line with your shoulders.** Twisting can lead to serious back injuries because when you move your shoulders first, your hips stay behind. Next time you need to pick up something or look behind you, move your hips first so your shoulders move in unison.

✔ **Keep your abdominal muscles pulled in.** Suck in your gut! Just as if you were tightening a belt, don't let your tummy muscles slacken for one minute. Use your breath to exhale, and pull in your abdominals with the tough part of a move and inhale slowly on the way back down.

Recruiting Your Upper Body for Core

Unlike your leg muscles, some of your upper-body muscles, like your biceps, are small muscle groups, so you want to avoid overtraining them. The triceps muscles are also made up of many different muscles located along the back of your arms. The biceps muscles work in opposition to the triceps, so working both muscle groups together is important to achieve balance and to keep the entire arm strong as you transition the following exercises through your core.

If you don't want to stand while doing the following exercises, you can use the exercise ball or a weight bench to sit on. However, of the two, I prefer using the ball because it challenges your balance and coordination as it increases your core strength when you're working with weights.

I suggest starting out with three to five pound hand weights; when you can comfortably, do this workout two to three times a week. Then work up to heavier dumbbells.

Just remember the following list of tips when using weights, to avoid injury:

✔ Keep your shoulders back and down.

✔ Keep your chest lifted.

✔ Keep your wrists in line with your elbows.

✔ Keep your hips in line with your shoulders.

✔ Keep your abdominal muscles pulled in.

Biceps curls

To do the biceps curl, you need three to five pound weights. As you gain strength, try using heavier dumbbells. The instability of the ball adds a new aspect of balancing to the biceps curl, making it more challenging for a better all-over workout.

To do this exercise, follow these steps:

1. **Stand with feet shoulder width apart. Hold your weights down by your sides, with your palms facing inward.**

2. **Pull in your abdominal muscles as you slowly bring your weights toward your shoulders (see Figure 13-1).**

   Your palms should be facing your shoulder.

   As you curl the weights toward your shoulders, concentrate on the biceps muscles. Doing so helps you isolate the movement and focus on the muscle that you're working.

3. **Hold for a few beats and then release the weights back to your sides.**

4. **Complete two sets of 10 to 15 repetitions.**

Follow these tips while doing this exercise:

- ✔ Keep a straight spine and pull in your abdominals while lifting the weights to your shoulders.
- ✔ Lower the weights slowly back to the starting position.

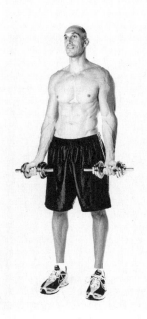 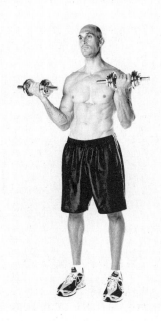

Figure 13-1:
Biceps
curls.

a   b

✔ Use a slow, controlled movement — don't jerk the weights up to your shoulders.

✔ Don't allow the elbow to shift forward or backward. Keep the upper arm as still as possible so only the elbow bends.

Alternating biceps curls

Beginners need three- to five-pound weights with the alternating biceps exercise. Advanced men and women can use heavier dumbbells.

To do this exercise, follow these steps:

1. **Sit on the ball with your feet shoulder width apart. Hold your weights down by your sides, with your palms facing inward.**

2. **Pull in the abdominal muscles as you slowly bring your right weight toward your right shoulder (see Figure 13-2).**

   Your palm should face inward toward the shoulder.

3. **Hold for a few beats and then release the weight back to your right side; repeat with your other arm.**

4. **Complete two sets of ten repetitions.**

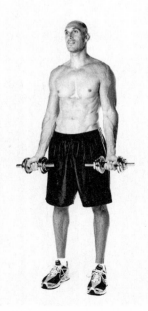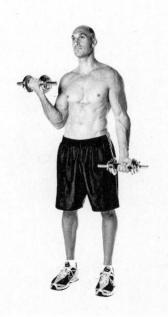

Figure 13-2:
Alternating
biceps
curls.

a   b

Here's what you need to remember for this exercise:

- ✔ Concentrate on your biceps muscle as you do this exercise.

- ✔ Contract your abs before lifting the weight to your shoulder.

- ✔ Use a slow, controlled movement — don't jerk the weights up to your shoulders.

Triceps press

The triceps press works the triceps (the back of the arms). Like with the biceps curl, this exercise is more challenging when you do it on the ball because you need to maintain your balance.

If you have a neck or shoulder injury, always check with your doctor first to see which exercises are appropriate for you.

Beginners need one three to five pound weight. Advanced ball users can use a heavier dumbbell.

To do this exercise, follow these steps:

1. **Sit on the ball with your feet shoulder width apart. Hold the weight in both hands, behind your head (as Figure 13-3a shows).**

   Keep your biceps next to your ears.

2. **Straighten your elbows, pressing the weight toward the ceiling (see Figure 13-3b).**

3. **Bend your elbows to slowly lower the weight behind your neck.**

4. **Complete two sets of ten repetitions.**

While performing the triceps press exercise, keep the following in mind:

- ✔ Hold the weight in both hands as you press up.

- ✔ Stare straight ahead and keep your neck long — don't let your head and neck tilt forward during this exercise.

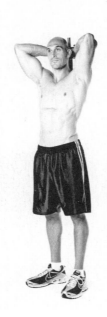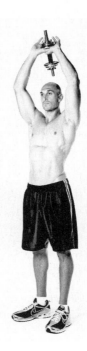

Figure 13-3:
Triceps
press.

a   b

Triceps kickbacks

To end the arm series, do some triceps kickbacks. You really need to pull in your abdominals before doing these movements.

To do this exercise, follow these steps:

1. **Step out into a lunge position, with your right leg forward and your left leg back.**

   Your left knee should be slightly bent.

2. **Holding your weights in your hands by your sides, keep your elbows bent at a 90-degree angle (as Figure 13-4a shows).**

3. **Moving only your forearm, extend your arms behind you until the elbow is straight (see Figure 13-4b).**

4. **Hold your weights back for a few seconds, and then return your arms to the starting position.**

5. **Complete ten repetitions and then switch legs. Increase repetitions when you feel comfortable.**

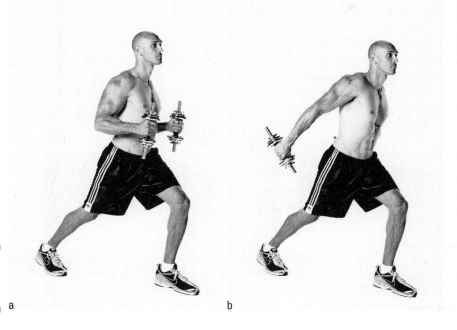

Figure 13-4:
Triceps
kickbacks.

a   b

To get the most out of this exercise, remember to:

✔ Keep your arms close to your sides while performing this exercise.

✔ Arch your back. Keep it straight and long as you lift your forearm behind you.

✔ Avoid letting your head drop down.

✔ Do keep your upper arm parallel to the floor.

Hammer curls

Seated hammer curls help develop good forearms. Don't be afraid to challenge yourself by increasing the weight as you go along to possibly a 15-pound or heavier dumbbell.

To do this exercise, follow these steps:

1. **Sit tall on the ball with your feet hip-distance apart. Hold your weights in your hands, with your palms facing each other and your arms down by your sides (as Figure 13-5a shows).**

2. **Bend your elbows as you bring your weights toward your shoulders with palms facing each other (see Figure 13-5b), keeping the abdominal muscles tight.**

   Be careful not to let the weights touch your shoulders.

3. **Slowly lower your weights, keeping tension on your biceps throughout the movement.**

4. **Complete two sets of 10 to 15 repetitions.**

You can really nail your biceps with the hammer curl exercise, if you remember the following tips:

✔ Keep your feet firmly planted on the floor, to keep the ball from moving.

✔ Keep your elbows from moving back and forth during this exercise.

✔ Use a slow and controlled movement throughout this exercise — don't release the weights too fast.

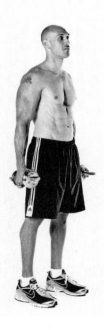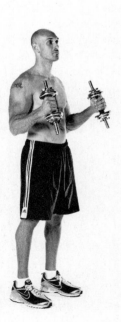

Figure 13-5: Hammer curls.

a   b

Bent-over rows

This exercise works the obliques, core, arms, and shoulders. Maintaining proper form throughout this exercise is important.

To do this exercise, follow these steps:

1. **Place your right knee on the ball, keeping your upper torso almost parallel to the floor.**

2. **Balance yourself by keeping your left hand on the ball and holding your weight in your right hand at your side (see Figure 13-6a).**

3. **Pull your weight up with a rowing motion as your elbow pulls back past your ribcage (as Figure 13-6b shows).**

   Be sure not to allow the shoulder to drop when pulling the elbow back.

4. **Hold for a few seconds, and then release the weight down to your side.**

5. **Complete ten repetitions. Then switch sides and repeat. Increase repetitions when you feel comfortable.**

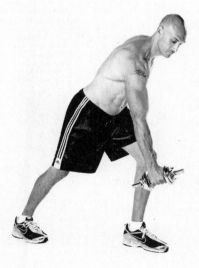 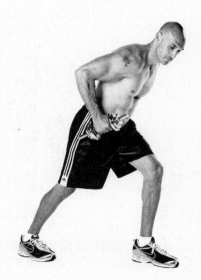

Figure 13-6: Standing rows.

a   b

While doing this exercise, remember to:

- ✔ Pull your elbow back as far as you can as you keep the shoulder blade squeezed back as far as possible toward the spine.

- ✔ Keep a long, straight spine during this exercise — don't lift your head because this movement causes your back to arch.

Body Resistance Core Series

Using the weight of your body as resistance to work against it is traditionally done with calisthenics. It's an extremely efficient way to build muscle and stay fit because it provides short bursts of intense training. You can work almost all muscle groups with only a few exercises.

Body weight resistance exercises are the perfect choice to do anytime because you don't to use extra weights to build great strength and lean muscle. Plus, they have many of their own benefits:

- ✔ You can do these exercises indoors or outdoors, without going to a gym or other facility for lifting weights.

- ✔ If you hate lifting weights, your body resistance training makes for an intense home exercise workout.

- ✔ Body resistance training improves cardiovascular endurance and core and muscular strength (because most of us weigh more than 100 pounds).

The following exercises challenge you in a different way than the other exercises in this book by using your own body weight. This is a good full-body workout you can do five times a week or as often as you feel comfortable.

Dips off a table

This exercise works your core as you strengthen your lower back and the muscles along the backs of your arms, the triceps.

Warning: Do not perform this exercise if you have any kind of shoulder injury.

1. **With your back facing the coffee table, bend your knees and place your hands behind you on the table. Place one leg on top of the opposite knee (as shown in Figure 13-7a).**

2. **Inhale as you bend your elbows and lower or dip your body down toward the floor. Exhale as you straighten your arms and press back up (as seen in Figure 13-7b).**

3. **Perform ten dips.**

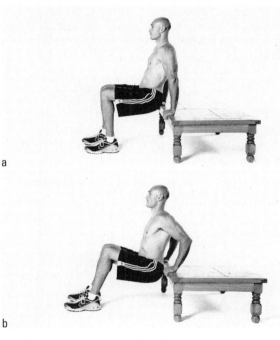

Figure 13-7:
Dips off a
table.

Get the most from doing dips by remembering to:

✔ Keep your elbows in and your arms close to your sides while performing this exercise.

✔ Avoid allowing your waist to drop below your knees, to prevent injury.

✔ Make your core and arms take over the workload — don't let your lower body do all the work.

Push-ups off a table

Doing a push-up off a table lends itself to working your core more intensely because you have to keep your lower back from dipping toward the floor and keep your spine long and straight. This exercise works your core, chest, arms, shoulders, and upper back.

To do this exercise, follow these steps:

1. **Stand facing your coffee table. Place your hands on the edge of the table for support as you straighten your arms and extend your legs back behind you (see Figure 13-8a).**

2. **Inhale as you lower your chest to the table in a classic push-up position by bending your elbows out to the side. Exhale as you press back up to your starting position (refer to Figure 13-8b).**

   Keep your back flat.

3. **Perform ten push-ups.**

While pushing through your push-ups, remember the following tips:

✔ Keep your elbows straight without allowing your elbows to lock as you press back into a push-up

✔ Don't arch your back or let your middle back dip toward the table.

✔ *Don't* let your head drop.

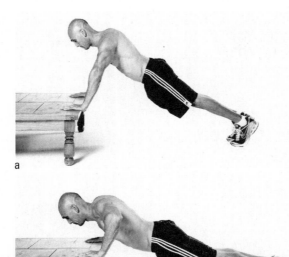

a

Figure 13-8:
Push-ups off
a table.

b

Squats

In this exercise, you work all the large muscle groups in the lower half of your body.

To do this exercise, follow these steps:

1. **With your arms out in front of you at chest level, lower in a squatting position so that your knees are parallel to the floor and keep your weight on your heels, not your toes (see Figure 13-9a).**

2. **Exhale as you press back up into a standing position, tightening your abdominal muscles (Figure 13-9b).**

3. **Perform ten squats.**

Here's what you need to remember for this exercise:

✔ Keep your abdominal muscles tight, to protect your back while doing this exercise.

✔ Keep your chest lifted and shoulders back throughout the entire exercise.

✔ Avoid strain on your knees by pressing through your heels.

✔ Avoid allowing your butt to drop below hip level. Remember, you're sitting down in a pretend chair, so you don't need to press back that far.

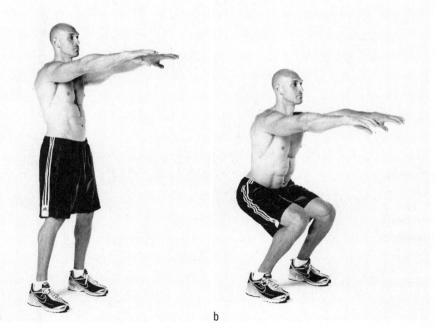

Figure 13-9:
Squats.
a   b

Walking lunges

Doing lunges from one side of the room to the other really calls on your core muscles to keep your chest lifted and shoulders back. This exercise strengthens your thighs and butt also.

To do this exercise, follow these steps:

1. **Take a big step forward with your right leg, and lower your right knee toward the floor as you lower into a lunge position (see Figure 13-10a).**

   Keep the stress off your knee by placing your weight in the heel of your front leg and not your toes.

2. **Perform five lunges to the opposite side of the room. Turn around and do five lunges back to the other side of the room.**

   You should finish exactly where you started (see Figure 13-10b).

Figure 13-10:
Walking
lunges.

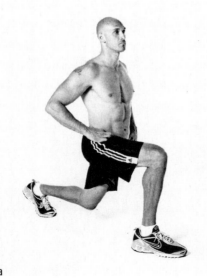
a

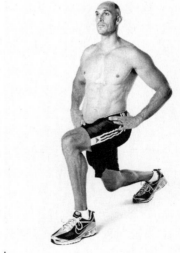
b

Hot muscles work better

Getting your heart rate up before you lift weights is essential because warming up your muscles and tendons increases your muscle elasticity (a muscle's length and its ability to stretch with heat), which enables you to handle heavier weights. Increasing your heart rate also helps you burn more calories during your workout.

You need only about five to ten minutes to increase your heart rate before your workout.

Taking a spin on a bike or a short jog on the treadmill does the trick. Jumping rope for a few minutes is also a good warm-up because it definitely gets your heart pumping in no time.

For another good way to warm up your body and have a little fun, see Chapter 4. You'll discover some great exercises that you can do to warm up your body properly before you head out the door for any kind of sport.

Remember these tips when you do this exercise:

- ✔ Keep your arms close to your sides or hands on your hips while performing this exercise.

- ✔ Keep your back straight and long as you point your tailbone toward the floor — don't arch your back.

- ✔ Keep your eyes lifted and your neck in line with your spine — don't let your head drop.

- ✔ Keep your front foot beyond your front knee as you keep your knee at a 90-degree angle.

Chapter 14

Core Stretches to Help Whittle Your Middle

In This Chapter

▶ Getting familiar with different stretches used to stretch your core

▶ Discovering the do's and don'ts of stretching your core

▶ Creating some functional stretches for your core to use every day

▶ Finding the best ways to stretch out your core

*Y*ou may have a strong back and sexy abs, but you still need to be able to touch your toes! So along with strengthening your core, you have to increase your flexibility. Stretching your core increases your flexibility by improving your range of motion. *Stretching For Dummies* (another book by yours truly and published by Wiley) can teach you how to stretch, and so can the core stretches in this chapter.

The stretches in this chapter target the abdominals, back, and waist, to help improve your range of motion. The combination of these stretches helps create a strong and flexible core. So first you stretch out your core, and then you strengthen it.

What to Do and What Not to Do

In Chapter 3 I talk about the basics of stretching and how it can help with your workout. You may want to review that section before moving on or take a peek at the following list as a refresher on just how important stretching really is:

✔ Stretch after your workout.

✔ Stretch a little bit every other day.

✔ Hold each stretch for 30 seconds.

✔ Avoid stretching until the point of pain.

✔ Stretch from the top to the bottom, down to the tip of your toes.

Abs and Back Core Stretch Series

I joke a lot in this book about getting a "six pack," but this series of stretches will really help you feel your abs. This series of core stretches will also work your back and all those other parts between your ribcage and your hips that make up your core.

Back extension

You see people every day who walk through life with rounded backs. You may even have this issue yourself. The back extension stretch is here to help you! This stretch is technically for the abdominals, but it's also great for the back muscles because it moves your spine in the opposite direction, giving the muscles a workout and increasing the mobility of your spine.

To do this stretch, follow these steps:

1. **Lie on your belly and prop yourself up with your elbows.**

   Your elbows should be directly under your shoulders. Lift yourself up out of your shoulders so that you aren't sinking into your shoulder blades.

2. **Inhale and, as you exhale, lengthen your spine and lift your chest as if you were going to move forward (see Figure 14-1).**

   While performing this stretch, imagine that you're trying to move forward but that your elbows and hips are glued to the floor and the space between each vertebra is increasing, lengthening your spine.

3. **Hold the stretch for 30 seconds or five or six slow, deep breaths.**

   You should feel this stretch in your abdominals.

Get the most from this stretch by remembering the following tips:

✔ Keep your neck long and in line with the rest of your spine.

✔ Pull your belly in toward your spine.

✔ Think of your chest moving forward and up — don't lift your chest toward the ceiling.

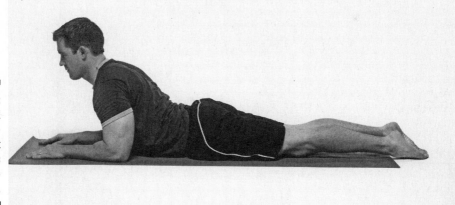

Figure 14-1:
The back extension that stretches the abdominals.

Step back and reach

This abdominal stretch is for the muscles that run along the front of your torso. Feel this stretch in your hip flexor, abdominals, and chest.

To do this stretch, follow these steps:

1. **Stand tall, with your feet together, your abdominals and chest lifted, your shoulders back, and your shoulder blades down (see Figure 14-2a).**

2. **Inhale and, as you exhale, lunge back with your left leg and reach your left arm over your head (see Figure 14-2b).**

3. **Hold this position for three deep breaths.**

4. **Inhale and bring your foot and arm back to starting position.**

5. **Repeat this exercise with your right leg and arm.**

6. **Repeat this stretch for six to eight repetitions, alternating sides (as in Step 5).**

   When you feel that you're ready to add a repetition or two, try doing two sets of six to eight repetitions.

Here are a few tips to remember while doing this stretch:

✔ Keep your spine long, even as you reach up and back down.

✔ Keep the motion slow and fluid, and use your abdominals to slow that motion.

✔ Avoid compressing your lower back as you reach up.

✔ Be sure that you don't twist or reach to the side.

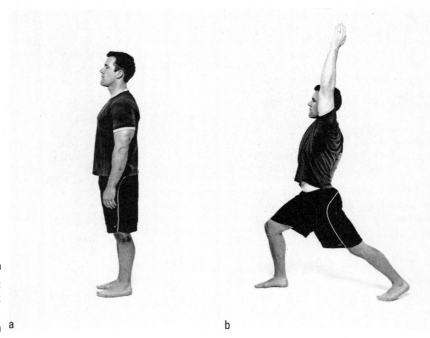

Figure 14-2:
Step back
and reach.

a   b

Side reach

This reach-and-stretch exercise is for the muscles that run along the outside of your hip, and the movements help your abdominals and your back. This stretch is a great daily stretch to keep you sitting tall and exercise good posture.

Perform this stretch by following these steps:

1. **Stand up tall, with your feet together, your abdominals and chest lifted, your shoulders back, and your shoulder blades down (see Figure 14-3a).**

2. **Inhale and, as you exhale, step out to the side with your right leg (side lunge), reaching your right arm overhead in the opposite direction (see Figure 14-3b).**

   The farther out you step to the side, the more you feel a stretch in your inner thigh, too.

3. **Hold the stretch for one deep breath.**

4. **Inhale and bring your body back to the starting position.**

5. **Repeat the steps on the left side.**

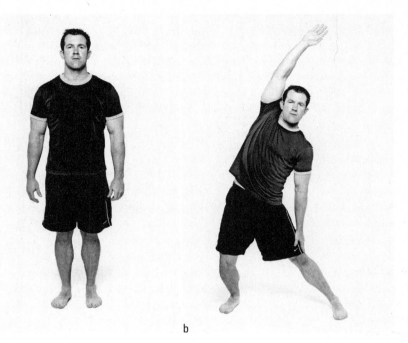

Figure 14-3:
Side reach.

a   b

6. **Repeat this stretch for six to eight repetitions, alternating sides (as in Step 5).**

   When you feel that you're ready to add a repetition or two, try doing two sets of six to eight repetitions.

Reach for great results with these tips:

- ✔ Keep your stationary leg straight so you feel the stretch in your inner thigh.
- ✔ Be sure that you don't twist or rotate your hips.
- ✔ Avoid bending forward as you lunge to the side.
- ✔ Do keep your weight back on the heel of the leg you step to the side with.

Lying spinal rotation

The lying spinal rotation is a good stretch to do when you want to stretch several muscles at once. In this stretch, you feel your back, oblique, neck, and chest muscles all stretch at the same time.

This stretch may be a bit uncomfortable at first, so always begin the stretch in your comfort zone for the first 10 to 15 seconds of the stretch, and then gradually increase the resistance of the stretch for the remainder. Never stretch beyond your pain threshold. Beginning slowly gives your muscles a chance to release and loosen up before you try to deepen the stretch.

This stretch involves the following steps:

1. **Lie on your back, with both legs extended and both arms extended out from your sides.**

2. **Exhale and raise your left knee to your chest, and slowly cross your knee over your body to the right (see Figure 14-4).**

3. **Turn your head to the left, or opposite direction, as you relax into the stretch.**

4. **Hold the stretch for 30 seconds; release the stretch, and repeat on the other side.**

You need to remember the following while performing this stretch:

✔ Breathe regularly as you hold the stretch.

✔ Progress through the stretch gradually.

✔ Be sure to not arch your back.

✔ Keep your shoulder blades on the floor rather than get your knee to touch the floor — don't force your knee to the floor.

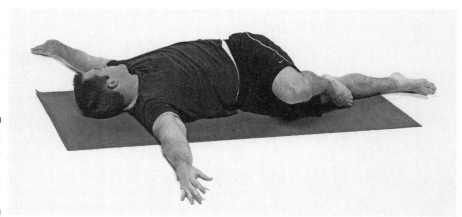

Figure 14-4:
How to perform lying spinal rotation.

Spinal rotation

A traditional stretch exists to stretch your buttocks, but by adding a spinal rotation to this buttocks stretch, you can stretch your back and buttocks at the same time. The two-in-one stretch can save you time and stretch your muscles more functionally.

To do this stretch, follow these steps:

1. **Stand up tall, with your right foot and right shoulder next to a chair, wall, fence, or other supportive surface for balance.**

2. **Lift your left foot and place your left ankle on top of your right thigh.**

3. **Inhale and, as you exhale, bend your right knee, and hinge or bend forward at your hips slightly so your hips move backward, similar to a squat (see Figure 14-5a for an example).**

4. **To deepen the stretch, grab hold of the chair or other supportive surface with both hands (see Figure 14-5b).**

5. **Hold the stretch for 30 seconds or five or six slow, deep breaths.**

6. **Repeat the steps on the other side.**

Figure 14-5:
Spinal
rotation for
the back
and
buttocks.

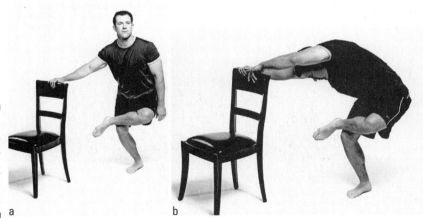

a   b

Why am I so sore after working out?

For decades, it was thought that the achy feeling you get after an intense workout was the result of a lactic acid build-up in the tissues of your muscles. Lactic acid is a normal by-product of the process of turning oxygen into energy, also known as *glycolysis.* When you work extra hard, your blood doesn't carry enough oxygen to wash your muscles clean of lactic acid and a residue builds up. Although many trainers may have told you your soreness was due to a lactic acid build-up in your muscles, soreness now has been attributed to tiny tears in the muscle fibers caused by the requirements of unfamiliar and excessive training. By helping to ensure that your muscles stay elastic and have a full range of motion in your joints, stretching can help protect you from those microscopic tears caused by newly intense levels of exercise.

While performing this stretch, be sure that you:

- ✔ Breathe regularly throughout the stretch.
- ✔ Tilt your pelvis back to feel a deeper stretch in your buttocks.
- ✔ Keep your knee directly above your ankle. Feel your weight mostly in your heel, not in your toes or the ball of your foot. Don't let your knee jut forward.
- ✔ Avoid bouncing or forcing the stretch.

Part V
Special Situations

The 5th Wave   By Rich Tennant

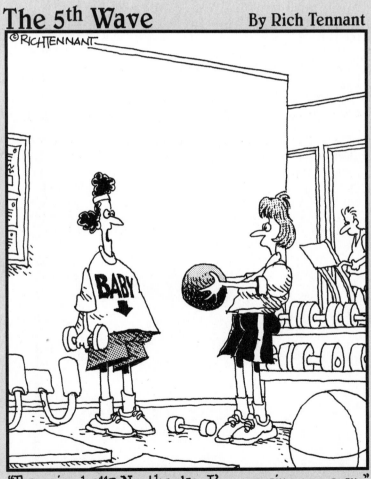

"Exercise ball? No thanks, I'm growing my own."

In this part . . .

In this part of the book, you discover that no matter what stage of life you're in, core exercises can improve your *daily* life. Chapter 15 focuses on pregnancy and postnatal core exercises to help you relax and strengthen your body in preparation of child birth and after. Chapter 16 gives you a series of fun exercises your kids can do to help them build basic core strength and learn the skills needed to stay fit for a lifetime. And finally, Chapter 18 contains core exercises that address the needs of anyone over the age of 60. If you're in one of these demographics, you'll find something suitable for you in this part!

Chapter 15

Pregnancy Moves for Your Core

∙∙∙

In This Chapter

▶ Core exercises that help you stay comfortable during pregnancy

▶ Using core-strengthening exercises to prepare your body for giving birth

▶ Knowing the benefits of working out during pregnancy

▶ Discovering exercises you can do with a growing girth

∙∙∙

*W*orking out during pregnancy is the best thing you can do for you and your baby. Many women — and doctors — find that exercising really helps relieve the discomforts of pregnancy. Just check out a couple of body benefits to exercising while you're pregnant:

✔ When you move your body on a daily basis and add some core-strengthening exercises, the pressure from your growing belly is relieved because your breathing becomes easier.

✔ Because your back muscles are engaged during core exercises, your posture improves, giving your baby more space to move around, as you're able to stand taller and lengthen your spine.

Within the last ten years, the medical profession has recognized the benefits of exercise for women during pregnancy. The challenges brought on by pregnancy and the stress of delivery are now countered with exercise to help women keep moving and stay strong throughout their pregnancies. In this chapter, I include some fun ideas to help keep you moving during your pregnancy and I include exercises that will also help keep you strong as your belly grows to alleviate the strain on your back.

At the end of this chapter, I cover some wonderful core exercises that you can use to strengthen your core and pelvic floor after giving birth and carrying around your baby for 9 months.

It's especially important to consult your doctor before starting an exercise program to become aware of the special demands placed on your body resulting from pregnancy for you and your baby.

Keeping a Strong Core with a Growing Belly

Because your center of gravity shifts during pregnancy and your belly usually greets people before you do, pregnancy can leave you feeling a bit off-center.

Support your growing belly and shifting body weight by helping take the pressure off your back and legs is the best thing you can do to help alleviate that uncomfortable feeling. Although many women would prefer to take pressure off their backs by simply lying down, you're better off giving your body the support it needs through some core moves. By supporting your lower back in different positions with some basic core exercises, you provide support that would otherwise be placed on the legs — which have way too much strain on them already.

Not only does exercise help you, by giving you a feeling of deep relaxation, but studies also show that working out during pregnancy increases your chances of having a faster and easier delivery and postpartum recovery.

When you get the urge to hit the couch instead of the gym while you're pregnant, just remember the following benefits you get from exercising during pregnancy:

- ✓ Alleviation of back pain, one of the biggest complaints that pregnant women have.

- ✓ Increased oxygen to the baby as a result of all the extra breathing that you're doing while exercising.

- ✓ Better digestion, which means help with morning sickness.

- ✓ Help with labor pains and preparation for delivery. (The stronger your muscles are, the easier your delivery will be because you'll be able to push harder.)

- ✓ Help with losing the baby weight and aids in a speedier recovery after delivery.

Giving birth has been compared to running a marathon, and that comparison is true — I know from experience! Being in great shape during your pregnancy helps ensure a healthier pregnancy and a faster recovery.

Kicking In Cardio for All Nine Months

You can choose from several good exercise options during your pregnancy. The following are ones you can do through all three trimesters, and that's why I recommend them highly. Read on to see my top three.

Walking

Walking is my recommended primary exercise during pregnancy, along with core moves and, of course, stretching (try *Stretching For Dummies* [Wiley], by yours truly). Walking helps to stretch the hip muscles while improving muscle tone in the pelvic floor and increasing circulation. Breaking up your walking routine can help boost your energy level by doing two shorter walks of 10 to 20 minutes a day instead of one longer one. And doing two shorter walks gives you a more workable routine that you can easily fit into your busy schedule. Of course, if you find yourself walking longer than ten minutes at a time, that's great, but remember to keep it simple and don't overdo it.

Swimming

For a complete pregnancy workout, try swimming. Being in the water leaves you feeling weightless, gets the heart pumping, and helps loosen those muscles. Swimming is just a great way to stay in touch with your body during pregnancy.

Moving

I'm not suggesting that you pick up and move your residence when you get pregnant. Instead, whatever you choose to do for exercise during pregnancy, just remember to keep moving. During the first trimester, you may find simply moving difficult because you feel tired and definitely need to take a catnap, which will help rejuvenate you throughout the day. Just try to keep up some form of simple exercise to keep that oxygen pumping to your growing baby and to help you stay fit during pregnancy. In other words, honor your body by listening to it: Rest when you need to and keep moving when you feel the desire!

Easing Discomfort with Core Moves

Core exercises can strengthen the abdominals even as your belly expands and help relieve tensions within your body from an overloaded back. Doing exercises that stretch out or round your back ease discomfort and help your muscles relax. The back roll-up exercise in this chapter and the chest and back stretch are two excellent ways to release built-up tension and discomfort from carrying around your extra weight.

Because of all the extra blood and fluids that your body is producing to support your growing baby, you may feel a buildup of pressure and a pulling sensation in your abdomen. The exercises in this section help counter these problems and many other discomforts you feel while pregnant.

Cat/cow

This move not only helps make your back feel better, but it also improves the range of motion in your spine, enhances strength and coordination of the muscles around your spine, and improves core muscle awareness in your entire back — all factors that make your lower back feel better and stay healthy.

To do this exercise, follow these steps:

1. **Get on the floor on your hands and knees, with your hands directly under your shoulders and your knees directly under your hips.**

2. **Inhale and arch your back, lifting your tailbone and eyes toward the ceiling (see Figure 15-1a).**

3. **Hold the stretch for a few seconds and then release the position back to neutral spine, and inhale again.**

4. **Exhale and contract your abdominals, rounding your back like an angry cat (see Figure 15-1b).**

5. **Hold this position for a few seconds and then release back to neutral spine.**

6. **Repeat this exercise four to six times.**

Get the most out of this exercise by

✔ Pulling your belly button toward your spine.

✔ Keeping the movement in your pelvis and lower back, not in your shoulders.

✔ Keeping your shoulders and neck relaxed — don't tense 'em up.

✔ Keeping your neck in a neutral position — don't overextend your neck while doing the old cow position.

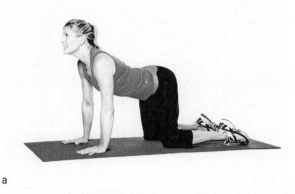

a

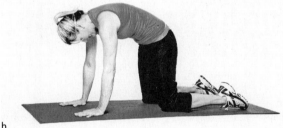

Figure 15-1:
Cat/cow.

b

Hip extension or kneeling bird/dog

This move is a good strengthening exercise for the abs, glutes, and lower back. Perfect for pregnancy!

To do this exercise, follow these steps:

1. **Kneeling on your hands and knees, place your hands below your shoulders and keep your knees directly beneath your hips (see Figure 15-2a).**

2. **Raise your right knee off the floor, extending your leg straight behind you, parallel to the floor, as you also extend your left arm straight out in front of you (as seen in Figure 15-2b). Hold for a count of three.**

3. **Lower your arm and leg back to the starting position, rounding your back like a cat.**

4. **Repeat this exercise, alternating sides, for ten repetitions for each side.**

Try to stay as relaxed as possible — don't tense up.

Here's what you need to remember for this exercise:

✔ Pull your belly button toward your spine.

✔ Avoid tensing your shoulders and neck.

✔ Use your diaphragm as you breathe to help you keep your balance and focus on keeping your spine completely neutral throughout this move.

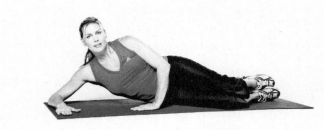

a

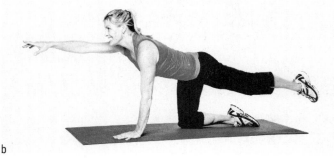

Figure 15-2:
Hip
extension
or kneeling
bird/dog.

b

Modified side plank

With a slight modification for pregnancy, the side plank works the core and includes the obliques. This exercise is one of the few you can do to directly help strengthen your abs during pregnancy.

To do this exercise, follow these steps:

1. **Start by lying on your side, with your bottom arm bent, legs straight, and feet staggered one in front of the other (as shown in Figure 15-3a).**

   Your elbow should be directly below your shoulder. Place your free hand on the floor in front of you or on your hip.

2. **Using your abs to lift your hips off the ground, keep your body as straight as possible (see Figure 15-3b). Hold for ten seconds.**

3. **Repeat one to three times and then switch sides.**

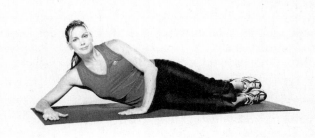

a

Figure 15-3:
Modified
side plank
pose.

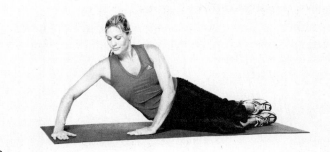

b

Remember the following tips while doing this exercise:

- ✔ Stagger your feet or place one in front of the other, to decrease the level of difficulty or just keep your knees and feet flat on the floor with knees bent at a 90-degree angle.

- ✔ Avoid tensing your shoulders and neck to keep them in a neutral, relaxed position.

- ✔ Keep your breathing steady — don't allow your hips to drop to the ground. Keep them in a straight line with your body from the shoulder down to your knees or feet.

Strengthening Your Stance with Standing Floor Moves

The next series helps build core strength while standing. It's important to maintain your balance throughout these exercises, so feel free to use the assistance of the wall if you need to steady yourself and keep from falling.

Side lunge

The side lunge uses the same technique as the forward lunge, except that you'll be stepping out at a 45-degree angle from the starting position instead of straight forward. It's good for strengthening your pelvic floor and working your abdominals plus all the major muscles in your lower body including the glutes, quads, hamstrings, and abductors/adductors.

To do this exercise, follow these steps:

1. **Standing with your feet about shoulder-width apart, keep your legs straight but not locked (see Figure 15-4a).**

2. **Take one large step sideways with your right leg. Slowly push back up, using your right leg and core muscles, to standing position (as shown in Figure 15-4b).**

3. **Alternate sides, doing ten reps on each leg.**

When you do side lunges, remember to

✔ Keep your hands on your hips as you step out sideways into a lunge.

✔ Keep your knees soft — don't lock your knees.

✔ Keep your breathing steady and strong — don't hold your breath.

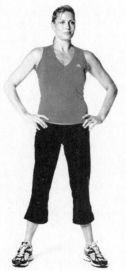 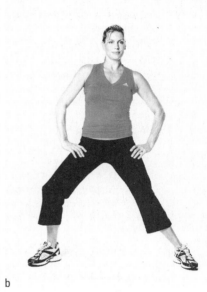

Figure 15-4:
Side lunge.

a   b

Who does the heavy lifting in your family?

It's tough to keep up with all the movements you have to do throughout the day: taking out the garbage, lifting your kids in and out of the car, bringing in the groceries from the car, and so on. The following tips will help reduce the risk of back pain when lifting and moving any kind of heavy weight:

- Tighten your stomach muscles before lifting.

- When standing, spread your feet shoulder width apart to give yourself a solid base of support, and then slightly bend your knees.

- Position the person or object close to your body before lifting.

- Lift with your leg muscles. Never lift an object by keeping your legs stiff while bending over it.

- Avoid twisting your body; instead, point your toes in the direction you want to move and pivot in that direction.

- When placing an object on a high shelf, move close to the shelf.

- During lifting movements, maintain the natural curve of your spine; don't bend at your waist.

- Do not try to lift something by yourself that is too heavy or that is an awkward shape. Get help.

Relieving Tight Muscles with Releasing

When you become pregnant, your body changes posturally so the baby can grow and your body can get ready for the birthing process. Increased hormones play a big part in these structural changes and allow your ligaments to loosen and stretch. You'll find that some of your muscles will tighten while others will loosen completely.

Releasing your back and abs provides you with these benefits during pregnancy:

- ✔ Aids in the circulation of all the extra blood you have pumping through your veins and arteries to various parts of the body
- ✔ Increases your energy level (a result of increased circulation)
- ✔ Reduces muscle tension in the lower back due to your growing belly
- ✔ Increases your range of movement in the joints
- ✔ Improves coordination (which you need desperately, thanks to your growing belly)

Given all those benefits, I like to include a few abdominal and back-releasing exercises to finish up a pregnancy core workout. With the flexibility exercises in this section, you can do some releasing for the muscles that get tight.

 Because you'll probably be doing a lot of sitting with your feet up during late pregnancy, take your time getting up from a seated position, to avoid standing up too quickly and getting dizzy.

Pregnancy core stretch

This stretch eases back pain and tension by targeting the whole muscle that extends from your neck to the small of your back. Be sure to do this stretch whenever you feel lower-back discomfort.

To do this exercise, follow these steps:

1. **Stand with your feet hip distance apart, keeping your knees relaxed (as shown in Figure 15-5a).**

2. **Holding on to a door or a chair for support, bend your knees and round your back, tucking your chin toward your chest and tucking your pelvis (see Figure 15-5b).**

3. **Hold for ten seconds and then repeat several times.**

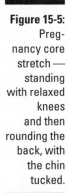

Figure 15-5:
Preg-
nancy core
stretch —
standing
with relaxed
knees
and then
rounding the
back, with
the chin
tucked.

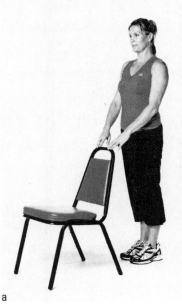 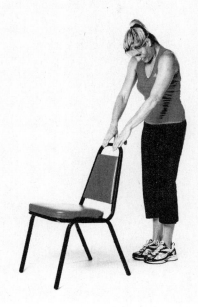

a   b

Remember these tips during this stretch:

✔ Hold on to something for balance during this stretch.

✔ Keep your knees slightly bent.

✔ Tuck your chin toward your chest, to stretch the entire back.

Chapter 16

New Mommy and Me Core Workout

· ·

In This Chapter

▶ Maximizing core exercises that help you bounce back after baby

▶ Using core-strengthening exercises to strengthen your pelvic floor and abdominals

▶ Reaping the rewards of starting early after giving birth

▶ Discovering exercises you can do with your baby in tow

▶ Bouncing back with your new little bundle of joy

· ·

Starting a fitness program for anyone can be daunting but it can be especially tough for new moms (and I speak from my own personal experiences). As the author of *Lose That Baby Fat* (M. Evans and Company, Inc.), I'm used to helping new moms start early to get back on the path to looking and feeling good about themselves again. And in this chapter, I not only lead you back to the path to looking and feeling good, but I also show you that getting back into exercise doesn't have to be so overwhelming, as long as you're armed with the proper tools.

In this chapter, I talk about finding the time to fit in exercise, and the importance of not overdoing it right after giving birth by setting realistic goals for yourself. I also show you some fantastic exercises where you can start incorporating your baby in your workout, which is beneficial to both of you. Mommy gets to fit in exercise and baby gets a little extra bonding time!

And of course, no mommy and me workout would be complete without a stroller to help you both get some fresh air and exercise while baby inevitably naps the moment you place him or her in the stroller! There are more tools and tips in this chapter so take advantage of the little time you have while baby's napping and read on.

Do's and Don'ts for New Moms

If you're committed to getting back in shape after having your baby, you can do several things to ensure your success. And, of course, you should also avoid some things at all costs to make sure you stay on the path to fitness. In the following sections, I give you some guidelines about what to do or not to do as you get back into exercising. Above all, remember that slow and steady does indeed win the race. So don't get discouraged — getting back into shape just takes time.

After your doctor gives you the go-ahead to exercise (around six weeks for vaginal births and eight weeks for cesarean sections) check out the following guidelines before you begin to make your transition a bit smoother for getting back in shape!

Do

Before you begin exercising postpartum, you definitely need to ensure that you

- **Set some goals.** You're more likely to stick with a program when you've set some goals for yourself, so write down your fitness goals.

- **Remember that you're not eating for two anymore!** Strive to eat a well-balanced diet that includes lots of fresh vegetables and fruit.

- **Eat several minimeals throughout the day, and don't go hungry.**

- **Keep your current fitness level in mind before starting your exercise program.** By doing so, you'll be able to establish goals that meet your specific needs.

- **Choose alternatives to satisfy your cravings, when possible.** Consider fat-free chocolate pudding over ice cream.

- **Always stretch before and after your exercise routine (try my book *Stretching For Dummies* [Wiley]).**

- **Increase slowly the intensity of your workouts over time as your stamina grows.** Trying to do too much at once will burn you out fast.

- **Partner up with another mom or friend.** You'll help motivate each other, and it's easier to stick to anything with a buddy.

- **Grab a healthy snack instead of eating junk food.** Try string cheese, raisins, nuts, carrots, crackers and peanut butter, and so on.

What is *diastasis recti?*

Ever heard or felt a separation in your abdominal wall? Better known as *diastasis recti,* it usually happens during the second or third trimester of pregnancy. This condition is painless but normal, although your doctor should check it out at your postpartum check-up before you begin exercising.

Here's what you'll find out if you have it:

If the split is more than three finger-widths, you'll need to avoid any twisting movements or spinal rotation. You can splint your abdomen with your hands or a towel during spinal flexion, until the split reduces to one finger-width or less. The biggest concern is that the intestines may be pushed out through the thin fascia and cause a hernia, which looks like a bulge under the skin. Persistent diastasis recti may be surgically corrected, usually at the time you have another baby.

Don't

For true fitness success after you have your baby, make sure that you don't

- ✔ **Do too much at once.** Your body needs time to recover, so take time to do so.

- ✔ **Skip breakfast.** Eating breakfast jump-starts your metabolism and provides you with the energy you need to get through the day.

- ✔ **Skip naps.** With a new baby, it's tough to get rest, let alone work out. Take catnaps for 10 to 20 minutes when you can — it really helps.

- ✔ **Set unrealistic goals.** A healthy rate of weight loss is one to two pounds per week. If you have 30 or so pounds to lose, don't expect it to come off overnight — you'll set yourself up for disappointment.

- ✔ **Compare yourself to others.** Everyone is different and, therefore, unique — what works for some may not work for others, and vice versa.

- ✔ **Be too hard on yourself.** It took nine months to grow a baby so give yourself time to get back to your former fitness level — be patient.

Kick-Starting Your Fitness Slowly with Kegels

I'm sure you know by now after giving birth, that there is nothing more incredible than the changes a woman's body undergoes during pregnancy. And just how shocking it is to look in the mirror after coming home from the hospital and still look six months pregnant! Although you may want to be active, exercise can be the farthest thing from your mind, right? You may feel overwhelmed or fatigued for the first three to six months after giving birth.

However, as the author of *Lose That Baby Fat* (M. Evans and Company, Inc.), I can tell you that working out early on in the postpartum period gives you back the energy you'll need to care for your new little one. It also helps clear the cobwebs from sleep deprivation. Plus studies have shown a relationship between starting physical activity after pregnancy and the decrease of postpartum depression, but only if the exercise is stress relieving and not stress provoking.

 Because you need stress-relieving exercise in your life, start off slowly with a few kegel exercises (strengthening exercises that rehabilitate and recondition the pelvic floor muscles) each day is a good way to get back in the mindset of exercise. You can perform kegels immediately after giving birth to help recondition the muscles and push out some of the water and fluids you'll be losing from the birth.

To do this move, follow these steps:

1. **Sit in a chair or lie down with your feet flat on the floor as you pull in the muscles you use to stop the flow of your urine.**

2. **Hold for three to five seconds before releasing and beginning again.**

After a few days of kegel exercises, begin the following series of exercises. Don't forget to work up slowly!

Warming Up to Your New Mom Workout

As a new mom, the challenges of finding any amount of time and the energy to exercise are tough. The following workout however is both effective and efficient. It should be done three times a week to begin and as you build in strength and stamina, you should increase the workout to five times a week.

Adding a stroller walk with your baby is the perfect compliment to the following exercises. So on the in between days or the days you're not doing this workout, you should try to walk with your baby in the stroller starting at 10 minutes and work your way up to a full 30 minutes when you can.

Before doing this new mom workout or any workout, you should warm up first to increase your circulation and get your blood pumping. I suggest five-to ten-minutes of low-level cardio to increase your core temperature and increase the flexibility of the muscles. Here are a few suggestions for warming up the body (if you have a few extra minutes to spare and want a really great warm-up, head to Chapter 4 for a few ideas):

✔ Walk on a treadmill for ten minutes at a slow to moderate pace.

✔ Jump rope for five minutes.

✔ Get on a stationary bike for ten minutes.

✔ Walk outdoors with your baby, starting with a slow pace and working up to a faster pace.

✔ Swim for half a mile.

Warming up your body increases the temperature of your muscles, which reduces the risk of injury.

Lying pelvic tilt

Pelvic tilts done lying down loosen up your hips and core area and get your circulation flowing so everything moves more freely. You can take your time with this movement — and don't forget to breathe!

To do this exercise, follow these steps:

1. **Lie on your back with your knees bent and feet flat on the floor. Make sure your spine is in the neutral position, and place your hands at your sides (see Figure 16-1a).**

2. **Slowly exhale as you roll your hips forward or toward the ceiling, until your lower back is pressed flat on the floor.**

3. **Inhale as you return to starting position, then roll your hips backward until your lower back arches slightly (see Figure 16-1b).**

4. **Repeat ten times.**

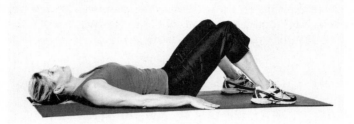

a

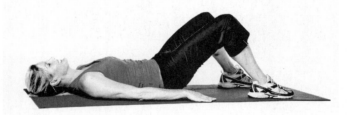

Figure 16-1:
Lying pelvic
tilts.

b

Make sure that you do the following with this exercise:

✔ Focus on moving just your lower back, not your thighs.

✔ Go only to the point of feeling good without straining — don't tilt or hold the movement too long.

✔ Keep your breathing steady and strong — don't hold your breath.

Beginning side plank

To do this exercise, follow these steps:

1. **Lie on your left side, propping up your body on your left elbow. Place your elbow directly beneath your shoulder. Bend both of your knees at a 90-degree angle, stacking your thighs on top of one another (see Figure 16-2a).**

   Place your right hand on the floor in front of your body for support. Ensure that your body from your head down to your toes is in a straight line, with a neutral spine.

2. **Lift your hips so that your torso comes off the ground and your body is in a straight line from your head to your knees. Try to hold this position for 15 to 30 seconds (see Figure 16-2b).**

3. **Repeat three times.**

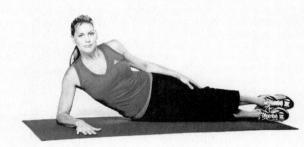

a

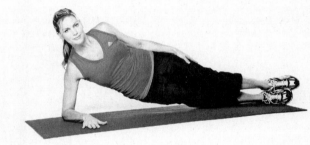

Figure 16-2:
Beginning
side plank.

b

With the side plank, remember to follow these tips:

 ✔ Pull in your abdominal muscles for support.

 ✔ Avoid letting your hips drop toward the ground.

 ✔ Keep your breathing steady and strong — don't hold your breath.

Postpartum bridge

The bridge — specifically, this postpartum version — works the hips, abdominals, and lower back, better known as your core. Be sure to use a smaller range of motion — don't lift your hips too high off the ground, to avoid stress on your lower back.

How fast should I lose the baby weight?

So what is realistic at this stage in the game? I've found that losing 2 pounds a week is realistic and safe (if you're breast-feeding, it's 2 ½ pounds a month). Two pounds a week ensures that the skin retracts or tightens and doesn't sag. And if you gained more than 35 pounds while you were pregnant, you need to allow an extra month of exercising and eating less or maintaining portion control for each additional 5 pounds of weight that you gained. So if you gained 45 pounds, you should achieve your goal and regain your pre-pregnancy weight around month nine or ten. Remember, it took nine months to grow your baby, so it will take at least that much time to regain your pre-pregnancy figure.

Most important of all, keep in mind that your ultimate goal is not only to lose the baby weight, but also to tone and tighten the areas that were stretched out during pregnancy and delivery.

To do this exercise, follow these steps:

1. **Lie flat on your back, with your knees bent and feet hip-width apart and flat on the floor. Place your hands on the floor at your sides. Keeping the spine neutral, pull your belly button in toward your spine (see Figure 16-3a).**

2. **Slowly lift your hips toward the ceiling, allowing your butt and lower back to lift up toward the ceiling and off the floor (see Figure 16-3b).**

   Hold for three to five seconds.

3. **Slowly lower your hips again, allowing your back to return to neutral position.**

4. **Repeat ten times.**

To avoid creating a bridge that gets you nowhere, keep these tips in mind:

✔ Pull in your abdominal muscles for support.

✔ Maintain a neutral spine.

✔ Breathe! Don't hold your breath.

Bicycle

Hands down, this exercise is my favorite for new moms because it targets the waist, obliques (muscles that run down the side of the waist), and abs. The twisting and pulling motion you do with your knees and upper body is perfect for getting your core back in shape fast!

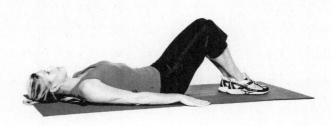

a

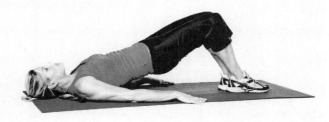

Figure 16-3:
Postpartum
bridge.

b

To do this exercise, follow these steps:

1. **Lie on your back with your knees bent and thighs perpendicular to the floor. Place your fingers just behind your ears (see Figure 16-4a).**

2. **Lift your shoulders off the floor as you straighten the right leg and bring the left knee in toward your right armpit. Without relaxing the torso or returning your shoulders to the floor, repeat on the other side by straightening the left leg and pulling the right knee in toward the left armpit (as shown in Figure 16-4b).**

3. **Alternate the legs in a slow bicycling movement 15 times on each side.**

Consider a few do's and don'ts for this exercise:

✔ Pull in your abdominal muscles for support.

✔ Avoid allowing your hips to drop toward the ground.

✔ Keep your breathing steady and strong — don't hold your breath.

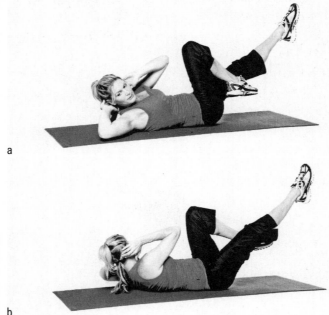

Figure 16-4:
Bicycle for a
great waist
and abs.

a

b

Crunch (postpartum)

The simplest way to regain strength in your core and endurance is to do crunches. However, you want to progress slowly. Consider a few ideas on how to do that:

- First try doing crunches with your arms outstretched, reaching your hands toward your knees.

- Second, try doing crunches with your arms across your chest (as shown here).

- Finally, you can do crunches with your hands placed behind your head and neck for support.

To do this exercise, follow these steps:

1. **Lie on your back, with your knees bent and hands crossed in front of your chest. Your feet should be flat on the ground (see Figure 16-5a).**

Be sure to keep a space between your chin and chest as you're looking up toward the ceiling.

2. **Raise your chest until your shoulder blades lift off the floor (as shown in Figure 16-5b).**

3. **Slowly lower back to the floor.**

4. **Repeat five to ten times, gradually progressing to more repetitions when you feel comfortable.**

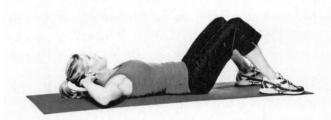

a

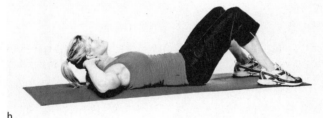

Figure 16-5:
Crunch
postpartum.

b

Get your crunch correct by following these tips:

✔ Don't use your hands and arms to help lift you; use your abdominals.

✔ Keep your abdominals pulled in toward your spine throughout the entire movement.

✔ Don't raise your head and shoulders more than just off the ground.

Push-up on knees

Push-ups on your knees are a good way to regain strength in your belly and core area. You can progress to push-ups on your toes as you get stronger, but always keep in mind that your back should remain straight and should not buckle from the weight of your body.

Keeping your knees on the ground with a towel beneath them will ease the harshness of the floor and provide more support for your joints.

To do this exercise, follow these steps:

1. **Kneel on your knees and place your hands shoulder-width apart on the floor in front of you (as shown in Figure 16-6a).**

   Make sure that your hands are directly below your shoulders on the floor.

2. **Lower the upper body toward the floor, bending your elbows out to the side (see Figure 16-6b).**

3. **Straighten your elbows and exhale as you press back up into starting position.**

4. **Complete ten repetitions.**

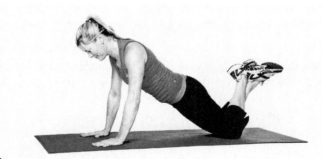

a

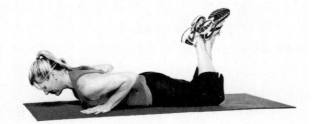

Figure 16-6:
Push-ups.

b

Here's what you need to remember for this exercise:

- ✔ Keep your abdominal muscles tight, to maintain your weight.

- ✔ Use proper breathing, inhaling as you lower and exhaling as you press back up.

- ✔ Keep your back straight and in line with your head and the rest of your body. Don't arch your back.

Mommy and Me Moves: Fun Stuff to Do with Your Baby

The following series of core exercises is so much fun to do with your baby. Finding time to work out after giving birth is so hard — now you have no excuse not to! Just grab a front baby carrier or a sling, and get to work with your little one.

Baby hip bridge

Hip bridges are so fun to do with your baby 'cause you get the interaction of looking at your little one as you use him for resistance! Your baby will love the slow up-and-down motion used in this exercise — and you'll feel the burn, too!

1. **Lie down on the floor with your knees bent and feet flat on the floor. Sit your baby on your hips, resting his back against your thighs. Gently hold him in position (shown in Figure 16-7a).**

   Be sure to engage your abs by pulling your belly button toward your spine, and press your weight down through your heels.

2. **Slowly lift your hips off the floor by squeezing your butt and engaging your abs (see Figure 16-7b). Your body should be in a straight line from your knees to your shoulders.**

3. **Slowly return to starting position.**

4. **Do 10 to 15 repetitions.**

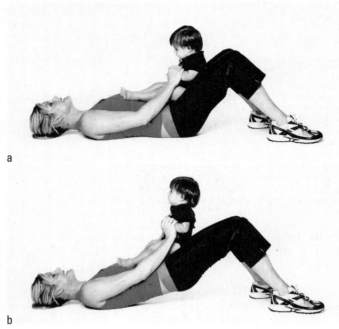

a

b

Figure 16-7:
Baby hip
bridge with
baby in lap.

Get hip to the following tips for this exercise:

- Make sure that your baby is totally secure during all movements.

- Try the movement without your baby first, to see if it's doable for you.

- Avoid letting your butt touch the ground in between lifts if you want to increase the level of difficulty.

Crunch with baby

Ah, yes, the ab crunch — another one of my favorite exercises to do with baby. You can play peek-a-boo as you lift your shoulders up and down off the floor in this exercise, and your baby will crave more — maybe before you do!

1. **Lie down on the floor or a mat with your knees bent and feet flat on the floor. Sit your baby on your hips, resting her back against your thighs. Gently hold her in this position (see Figure 16-8a).**

   Engage your abs by pulling your belly button toward your spine.

2. **Hold on to your baby and raise your chest until your shoulder blades lift off the floor (see Figure 16-8b).**

3. **Slowly lower back to the floor.**

4. **Complete 10 to 15 repetitions.**

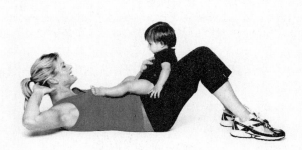

a

Figure 16-8:
Crunch with
baby.

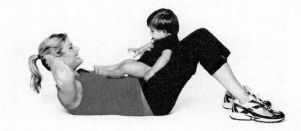

b

While doing crunches with your baby, be sure to follow these tips:

✔ Keep one hand on your baby at all times.

✔ Stop this exercise if it feels too strenuous.

✔ Avoid raising your shoulders off the ground more than just slightly.

Reverse crunch with baby

I also call this the airplane exercise because when you put your baby on your shins, you can gently roll from side to side like an airplane with wings. It's a fun exercise to do and a great core workout when you lift your baby up and down using his weight for resistance.

To do this exercise, follow these steps:

1. **Lay your baby prone (belly down) on your shins so they're facing you while you lie on your back. Hold on to your baby with your hands to keep him secure (see Figure 16-9a).**

2. **Keeping your knees bent and your feet off the floor, engage your abdominal muscles by pulling your belly button in toward your spine.**

3. **Pull your knees toward your chest, focusing on your abdominals as you hold on to your baby tightly in an airplane position (see Figure 16-9b).**

4. **Slowly lower your hips and legs back to the starting position, to complete one rep.**

5. **Aim for one to three sets of 10 to 15 repetitions.**

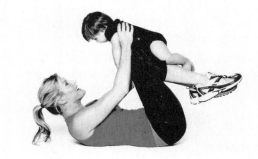

a

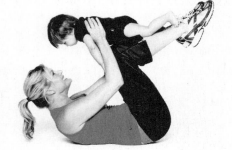

Figure 16-9:
Reverse
crunch with
baby.

b

For this exercise, remember to do the following:

- ✔ Make sure that baby is totally secure in all movements.
- ✔ Start out very slow, lifting your shins only slightly.
- ✔ Keep the pace slow and steady — don't lose control of the motion or use momentum.

Plank with baby

The plank with your baby lying underneath you really makes you work your core because you won't want to fall on your baby! Be sure to stay strong and lifted, and maintain a long, straight back during this exercise.

Be sure to stay lifted during the plank exercise so you don't fall on the baby. If you don't feel strong enough yet to support your full body weight, just keep your knees on the floor and straighten your forearms.

To do this exercise, follow these steps:

1. **Kneeling over your baby with your knees and forearms on the floor, keep your elbows directly below your shoulders. Your feet should be touching or no more than an inch apart.**

2. **Lift your body on your forearms and toes, keeping your body as straight as possible. Maintain this position for as long as possible; challenge yourself as you build up to longer periods in the plank position (see Figure 16-10).**

3. **Hold the position for 10 to 15 seconds in the beginning, working your way up until you can hold the position for longer.**

Not only should you avoid pooping out while doing the plank, but you should also remember these tips:

✔ Keep your back long and straight.

✔ Avoid allowing your hips or knees to drop toward the floor.

✔ Breathe steady and engage your abs.

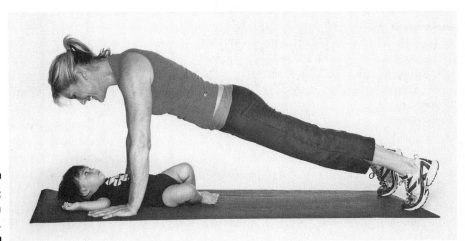

Figure 16-10:
Plank with baby.

Lunge with baby in carrier

This exercise uses a front baby carrier or sling. Plus, you can hold on to a wall or chair for additional balance, if you need to. Lunges work to strengthen your core, butt, and hips as you press back up to a standing position. Adding the weight of your baby makes for great resistance and a more intense workout.

To do this exercise, follow these steps:

1. **Standing tall with your abs engaged to support you and your baby, step your right leg forward and left leg back so there's a wide distance between your feet (see Figure 16-11a).**

2. **Lower toward the floor by bending both knees. Your front knee should bend at a 90-degree angle with the ankle directly below it. Your back knee should lower straight down toward the floor (as shown in Figure 16-11b).**

3. **Push back up to the starting position to complete one rep.**

4. **Complete 10 to 15 repetitions on each side.**

Figure 16-11:
Lunge with baby.

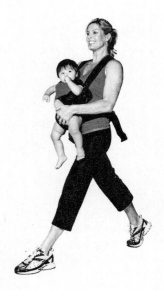
a

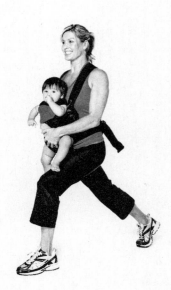
b

Remember these hints for this exercise:

- Keep your movements straight up and down — don't lean forward while lunging.
- Widen the stance between your legs if you have trouble maintaining your balance.

Plie squat with baby

Plies are a great way to strengthen your core and abdominals, and tighten up your inner thighs. Because safety should always be your main concern for you and your baby, make sure that your baby is totally secure in all movements. If any exercise is too strenuous with your baby, try it without her.

To do this exercise, follow these steps:

1. **Stand with your feet wider than shoulder-width apart and your knees slightly bent, with your toes turned outward (see Figure 16-12a).**

   Make sure your knees and toes are pointing in the same direction. Engage your abs by pulling them in and standing tall.

2. **Press straight down until your thighs are almost parallel to the floor (as shown in Figure 16-12b).**

   Make sure your knees don't reach past your toes.

3. **Squeeze your butt as you straighten your legs back to starting position, to complete one rep.**

4. **Complete 10 to 15 repetitions.**

Plie away with these tips:

- Keep your knees pressed out, to strengthen your inner thighs even more.
- Keep your toes pointed forward at all times.
- Keep your spine straight and long — don't lean forward.

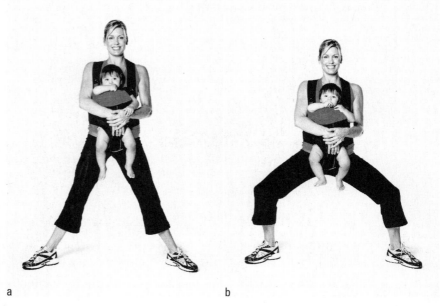

Figure 16-12:
Plie squat
with baby.

a   b

Squat with baby

This exercise uses a front baby carrier, or you can hold your baby securely in your arms. Safety should always be your main concern, so make sure that your baby is totally secure in all of the following movements. Using the weight resistance of your baby makes the squat more intense and helps you get a better rear view!

To do this exercise, follow these steps:

1. **Stand with your feet wider than shoulder-width apart. Toes and knees should be pointing forward. Engage your abdominals and stand tall.**

2. **Slowly lower your butt toward the ground and bend at your hips as if you were going to sit back in a chair. Keep your weight in your heels and your back as upright as possible (see Figure 16-13a).**

3. **Straighten your legs and come back up to the starting position (refer to Figure 16-13b).**

4. **Complete 10 to 15 repetitions.**

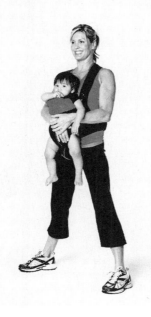
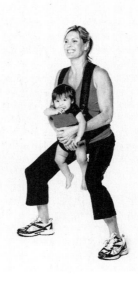

Figure 16-13:
Squat with
baby.

a   b

Squat safely and effectively by following these tips:

- ✔ Keep your knees soft — don't lock them.
- ✔ Keep your baby in an upright position as you squat.
- ✔ Stop if you feel pain in your knees.
- ✔ Hold on to a chair to help maintain your balance throughout the movement.

What's in a core?

What people used to refer to as their midsection is now better known as the core. Your core is made up of the deep abdominal and back muscles that work as stabilizers for the entire body. These muscles are referred to as "deep" muscles because you can't see them. Still, these muscles are responsible for maintaining the body's core stability.

The three muscles in the core, or midsection or trunk, of the body are the *transverse abdominus, multifidus,* and *quadratus lumborum.* These muscles work together to protect the spine and to help with everyday activities, such as lifting, throwing, bending, reaching, and running. So you can see why keeping the stabilizer muscles well conditioned is extremely important.

Chapter 17

Exercises for Kids to Help Build Core Strength

Kids are like mini video cameras — they imitate everything they see. My two-year-old always seems to find my weights, no matter where I put them, and drags them out to play. My friend suggested that instead of trying on my shoes, my daughter plays with my fitness equipment because they are my tools — she sees me exercising so she wants to exercise, too. So exercising in front of your kids sets a good, healthy example that they can follow. However, you don't really want your five-year-old training with you for that triathlon coming up next summer — such training is a bit much (okay, a lot much!) for a youngster, but core training is perfectly adaptable and positively fun for children to do.

In this chapter, I offer a few exercises kids love to do that will help them acquire the basic skills needed to exercise and play sports. The exercises in this chapter also help them build a strong back and develop good abdominal muscles for life! Because children are naturally active no matter where they are (especially in the car), it's important to encourage them to enjoy exercise and have fun doing it whether they're at the beach or right in your own backyard. Parents can help by getting children involved in fitness at a young age. It really is one of the best things you can do to establish a lifetime of healthy activity.

Parents, I assure you this workout is anything but a waste of time for you. Many of the exercises I include in this chapter for your kids I also use for adult workouts in other sections of this book. With a little modification (speeding things up a bit), you can get a great workout and have so much more fun doing it alongside your kids. And maybe your kids will even challenge you to try something new and fun. I also designed the last two exercises in this chapter to be done with a partner, which makes them even more fun and challenging for children. Pairing up with brothers and sisters, cousins, and yes — even parents, helps to not only pass the time but, more importantly, gets everybody in good shape while they're having fun. What a great message to send to your kids and to reinforce for yourself: that doing things together, even exercising, can be fun as well as help you and your family reap the benefits of good health that will last a lifetime.

Getting the Facts on Kids' Fitness

Here are some facts and guidelines from the American Academy of Pediatrics:

- ✔ Kids should get no more than two hours of television or computer time a day.

- ✔ Boys should take 13,000 steps a day while girls should take 11,000.

- ✔ For children 7 to 12 year olds who did not meet the recommendations, they were three to four times more likely to be overweight than the other children in their class and age category who met the guidelines.

The following are tips and guidelines from the IDEA Health and Fitness Association on what your kids should be doing at different ages to help parents get children involved in exercise at any age:

- ✔ **Children ages two to five** need to learn basic movements and skills such as:

    - Catching

    - Rolling

    - Bouncing

    - Kicking

    - Tossing a ball

    - Running

    - Hopping

    - Skipping

    - Pedaling a tricycle

    - Galloping

✔ **Children ages five to seven:** At this age, children should be using basic motor skills that help build complex movements like hitting a ball with a bat and jumping over some stationary objects. They can also play harder and longer that younger kids which means they are now able to improve their level of fitness. Children at this age may become interested in team or group sports but not at a competitive level.

✔ **For children ages 8 to 12:** Children at this age can now participate in team sports more effectively and continue to grow in their fitness level. However, kids at this age lack the hormones needed for large muscle development. A decline in kids' activity usually begins at this age due to puberty and a feeling of self-consciousness when other kids start developing at different rates. Some different activities are walking a mile and keeping a log book of how fast they go, and strength training under the correct supervision. Building a strong body improves a child's self-esteem at this age and helps improve their attitude.

✔ **For children ages 10 to 12:** Children at this age continue team sports and group activities as well as begin to participate in individual activities like swimming, skating, and walking. Major hormonal changes are occurring, which make children feel awkward both physically and socially, determining what activities they become involved in. Best to look for classes that focus on varying levels of development like beginner, intermediate, and advanced rather than chronological age because of the different rates of maturity that are occurring.

Taking in Some Tips on Working Out with Your Kid

Most kids like to really go for it when they first try something new — like throwing themselves down a slide at break-neck speed or riding their bike down a hill! You have to love and admire that kind of enthusiasm. However, you have to rein in that enthusiasm until you're confident that your kids are safely performing each move. In the spirit of making things go as smoothly as possible the first time out, here are a few important workout tips that you and your kids need to know before they get started:

✔ **Make sure you monitor your kids** the first few times they try the exercises until you feel confident they are using proper form and get the hang of it.

✔ **Make sure that your kids follow the instructions** in this chapter thoroughly.

✔ **Be sure they use a slow and steady motion** when doing each exercise until they become pros at it — which, for kids, means at least once or twice because they pick things up so much quicker than we do!

✔ **Make sure they don't hold their breath** during the exercises. Holding their breath won't help them perform the exercises any better and will only leave their little lungs short of oxygen!

✔ **Have them perform each exercise without straining or injuring themselves.**

Working Your Kid's Core

The following exercises are fun moves your kids can do to help them develop some basic skills and start building core strength. You can do these moves with your kids or just watch them to make sure they're performing them correctly the first few times. Be sure to do the following exercises wherever you have enough space to move around...in your living room or even better, outside while you get some fresh air.

Froggy jumps

Although the object of this exercise is to warm up your entire body at once, this exercise comes with a bonus — at least for parents. Kids love this exercise, and they love to do it outside. So kids can jump the entire length of the backyard and be ready to go to bed early! To do this exercise, follow these steps:

1. **Stand with feet hip-width apart and crouch down, bending your knees out to the side (as shown in Figure 17-1a).**

   Place your hands on the floor in front of you for support.

2. **Jump up pushing through your heels like a frog, using your hands for an extra push.**

   Be sure to straighten your legs fully at the top of the jump (refer to Figure 17-1b).

3. **Return your heels and hands back down to starting position before beginning another froggy jump.**

   Complete 10 to 15 repetitions.

Try traveling or moving across the floor and back doing froggy jumps.

When you do this exercise, remember to

✔ Keep your back straight as you jump up in the air.

✔ Avoid hunching over while you jump.

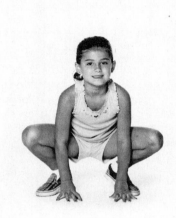
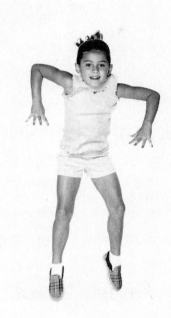

Figure 17-1:
Froggy
jumps.

a   b

Jumping jacks

Jumping jacks are a great way to warm up your core and strengthen it. By lifting your arms above your head and lowering them back down, you get a nice workout for your back and waist along with your abdominals and shoulders.

To do this exercise, follow these steps:

1. **Stand tall with your feet together and arms down by your sides. Jump your legs shoulder-width apart as you raise your arms above your head (as shown in Figure 17-2a).**

2. **Jump your legs back together as you bring your arms back down along your sides (refer to Figure 17-2b).**

3. **Jump to the rhythm — out, in, out, in, out, in.**

   Repeat for 10 to 15 repetitions.

Here are some things to keep mind for this exercise:

✔ Straighten your legs as you jump in and out.

✔ Keep your knees soft and unlocked — don't lock your knees.

✔ Keep the rhythm — in, out, in, out. Don't let your arms and legs get out of sync with each other.

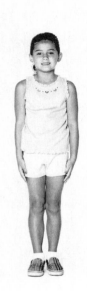
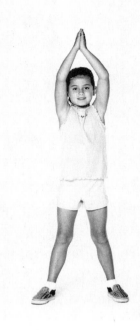

Figure 17-2:
Jumping
jacks.

a   b

Push-ups on knees

Push-ups on your knees are a good way to gain strength in your belly and core area. (Using a mat or towel helps to cushion knees from the ground.) Kids can progress to push-ups with straight legs as they get stronger.

Whenever adults or kids do push-ups with straight legs, their back should remain straight and not buckle in or dip from their body weight.

To do this exercise, follow these steps:

1. **Kneel on your knees and place your hands a little wider than shoulder width on the floor in front of you (as shown in Figure 17-3a).**

   Make sure that your hands are directly below your shoulders on the floor.

2. **Lower toward the floor with the upper body, bending your elbows out to the side (see Figure 17-3b).**

   Try leading with your chest instead of your head or hips to make the move easier.

3. **Straighten your elbows and exhale as you press back up into starting position.**

   Complete ten repetitions.

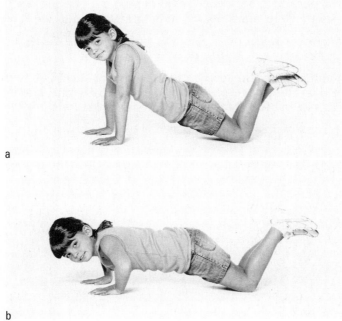

a

Figure 17-3:
Push-ups.

b

You can perform proper push-ups when you:

- ✔ Keep your abdominal muscles tight to help you maintain your weight and keep your back from sagging.

- ✔ Use proper breathing, inhaling as you lower and exhaling as you press back up.

- ✔ Keep your back straight and in line with your head and the rest of your body — don't arch your back.

- ✔ Don't allow your head to drop or look up to keep your neck in proper alignment with the rest of your body.

Bicycles

Bicycles are the best exercise to work your abs or tummy muscles. The twisting and pulling motion you do with your knees and upper body is perfect for getting your core in shape fast and is a lot of fun for kids and adults to do.

To do this exercise, follow these steps:

1. Lie on your back with your knees bent and thighs perpendicular to the floor. Place your fingers just behind your ears (see Figure 17-4a).

2. Lift your shoulders off the floor as you straighten the right leg and bring the left knee in toward your right armpit.

3. Without relaxing the torso or returning your shoulders to the floor, repeat on the other side by straightening the left leg and pulling the right knee in toward the left armpit (as shown in Figure 17-4b).

4. Alternate the legs in a slow bicycling movement ten times on each side.

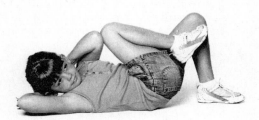

a

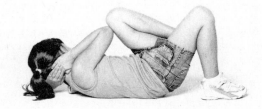

Figure 17-4:
Bicycle for
strong abs.

b

Pedal your way to success by following these tips:

✔ Pull your abdominal muscles in for support.

✔ Allow your hips to drop down toward the ground by keeping your abs tight — don't arch you back.

✔ Keep your breathing steady and strong — don't hold your breath.

✔ Keep your elbows pointed out to the side — make sure that you don't allow your elbows to pull forward.

Pairing Up for Exercise — Family Style

The next two exercises are extra fun because you do them with a play date, sibling, or parent. You'll see how fun it is for all your family members to sit on each other's feet and cheer them on as you try the following paired-up exercises. You can even make a little game out of these exercises by setting up a little circuit in your backyard like the following:

1. **Do some jumping jacks to warm up your body.**

2. **Move onto ball passing for one minute.**

3. **End with sit-ups holding each others' feet for one minute.**

Ball passing

Ball passing is a good way to help tighten your tummy muscles as you pass the ball back and forth between each other. This exercise also teaches the importance of teamwork, an important skill that everyone needs to take advantage of.

To do this exercise, follow these steps:

1. **Stand across from your partner a little farther than arms' length away.**

2. **Using both your hands, pass a volleyball, basketball, soccer ball, or any ball that can be passed comfortably between you and your partner at chest level (as shown in Figure 17-5a).**

   Remember to pass the ball — not throw it hard — at your partner!

   The ball will be at chest level when you are passing it between each other.

3. **Keeping your feet planted on the floor, continue passing the ball back and forth in a smooth fashion (refer to Figure 17-5b).**

   Complete 10 to 15 repetitions.

Try not to forget these important tips while passing the ball:

- ✔ Use your tummy muscles to pass the ball back and forth.

- ✔ Keep your back straight and stand tall — don't let your back arch away.

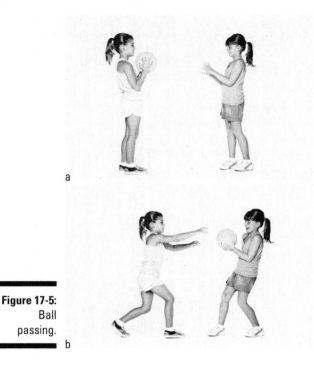

Figure 17-5:
Ball
passing.

b

Sit-ups: holding feet

These sit-ups work your tummy and back muscles and build strength in your legs. Sit-ups can be more fun to do if you count them out loud as you're performing them so it feels like you're coaching your partner through the exercise instead of just counting.

Pairing up different age groups for this exercise is fun because you can make a contest out of the exercise by seeing who can do the most sit-ups. Sometimes it's a little easier to have someone older than you hold your ankles or sit on your feet too.

To do this exercise, follow these steps:

1. **Lie on the floor with your knees bent and feet flat on the floor as your partner holds your ankles or tops of your feet down (as Figure 17-6a shows).**

    Your hands will be behind your ears with your elbows pointing out to the sides to support your neck.

2. **Tightening your stomach muscles, sit up straight and hold for a few seconds before returning back down to the floor (refer to Figure 17-6b).**

3. **Lie back down with a flat back completely on the ground before beginning the movement again.**

   Complete 10 to 15 repetitions.

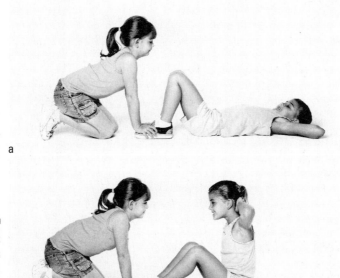

a

b

Figure 17-6:
Sit-ups
holding
each other's
feet.

Follow these tips for sit-up success:

✔ Use an exercise mat to cushion your back.

✔ Keep your head supported with your hands when you perform the sit-up; otherwise, you risk straining your neck.

Chapter 18

Seniors Taking the Core Challenge

In This Chapter

▶ Figuring out your core exercise limitations

▶ Understanding guidelines on exercise as you age

▶ Determining the right amount of weight for core-strengthening exercises

▶ Knowing the right forms of exercise you need to stay fit and healthy

*P*eople over age 65 represent the most rapidly growing group in the population (yes, baby boomers!), and the degrees of health and fitness of the people in this age group vary wildly. Nevertheless, when it comes to exercising and keeping a strong core, it is essential for seniors to strengthen the core muscles to help prevent falls and maintain independence throughout the senior years. Exercise is a powerful tool that helps the body and mind stay forever young. Plus, research has proven that strengthening the core muscles of the body through specific core exercises can help decrease injuries and help maintain strength and stamina for a lifetime, which means, you *don't* have to give in to aging any way but gracefully — and that's good news, isn't it?

Regular exercise is without a doubt one of the most important things you can do to keep your body functioning as smoothly as possible. It can't turn back the clock, but it can slow it down considerably.

Protecting Yourself with Exercise As You Age

Although you can do a lot to help make your life more active and easier as you age, the first and foremost is exercising. You need to do the following four specific types of exercise to stay young:

✔ **Endurance:** Exercises such as walking, speed walking, jogging lightly, swimming, or biking increase your heart rate, which helps build a strong heart and increases your stamina. Always start gradually, with only five minutes of any new activity at a given time until you work your way up to a full 30 minutes.

✔ **Strength:** Building your muscles increases your bone density and your metabolism, which is especially important for older adults because it not only helps to keep your weight down but also helps keep your blood sugar levels under control, which increase as you age.

✔ **Balance:** Building strong lower body and leg muscles helps prevent falls. Fractured knees, hips, and ankle joints become common as you age because bone mass begins to decrease. Working on your balance can help you from falling and prevent injuries.

✔ **Stretching:** Stretching allows you more freedom of movement as you age. The more freely you move, the better quality of life you'll have so you can remain independent in your golden years. For even more information on stretching, check out my other book, *Stretching For Dummies* (Wiley).

Exercising Safely As a Senior

Although you want your workouts to be challenging, you want to challenge yourself moderately to ensure that you're working out safely. To keep yourself challenged but safe while exercising, follow these guidelines:

✔ **Talk to your doctor first.** As with any new form of exercise, consult your doctor before you begin a workout program. Seniors with certain conditions, such as diabetes and coronary heart disease, may have to take a *Graded Exercise Test* (GXT) in which they get on a stationary bicycle or treadmill while their physician monitors their blood pressure and heart rate.

✔ **Do moderate workouts for 30 to 60 minutes at least twice a week on nonconsecutive days.** The American College of Sports Medicine suggests that seniors should follow this guideline, which basically means making sure that you have at least one full day of rest between workout sessions.

✔ **Target all your major muscle groups during your twice-weekly workouts.**

✔ **Do 10 to 15 repetitions of each exercise using a moderate level of intensity.** A moderate level of intensity equals 70 percent of the amount of weight you can lift in a single effort. Making a 70 percent effort in your workout should feel challenging but not exhausting to your muscles or require labored breathing. In other words, exercising shouldn't be painful in any way.

✔ **Begin gradually and increase the number of repetitions over time as you get stronger.** Because seniors are more prone to health concerns when working out, begin gradually using small movements with whatever exercise you choose to do and stop immediately if you feel fatigued or short of breath. Of course, for seniors who are severely out of shape, the less-is-more approach is always better because you can strain muscles and injure yourself by overdoing it.

Tuning In to Training Guidelines for Seniors

When it comes to strength training as you age, you should follow these guidelines to ensure your workouts are safe as well as effective:

- ✔ **Using weights or not:** Depending on your level of fitness, it's perfectly fine to start with no weights at all. Because starting with weights that are too heavy can cause injuries, using the resistance of your own body weight is a great way to start. As you build your strength and stamina, you'll be able to progress to using weights — but do it gradually. Keep in mind, slow and steady wins the race!

- ✔ **Adding weight:** When you do begin adding weights to your strength workout, add a challenging amount of weight gradually. Just enough that you feel like you're working out a bit harder than you were previously, because if you don't challenge your muscles, you won't get any stronger. Using one- to two-pound weights as you grow in strength and build a little muscle is a good way to enhance any strengthening program as your body adapts to the exercises.

- ✔ **Getting the timing right:** When you do begin lifting, use a slow three seconds to push your weight into place. Hold the position for only one second before taking three seconds to lower the weight back down to starting. And never let your weight drop! If you lower it slowly, you'll get the maximum benefit and see your muscles grow stronger faster because that's where the growth in the muscle takes place — on the downward part of the movement.

- ✔ **Adjusting your weight:** It shouldn't feel very hard to push your weight into place, but at the same time it should feel challenging. This part of the exercise is where listening to your body comes in handy. Stay in tune to what you're doing and feeling throughout your workout so you can make adjustments in the amount of weight you're using.

  The rule of thumb is: If you can't lift your weight eight times in a row, then it's too heavy and you should reduce the amount of weight you're using. However, if you can lift the weight more than 15 times in a row, then it's way too light for you so you need to increase the amount of weight you're using.

- ✔ **Doing reps and sets:** After you've determined the right amount of weight that's right for you, complete 8 to 15 repetitions in a row and then wait one minute before doing another set of 8 to 15 repetitions of the same exercise.

Always work up slowly and stop immediately if you feel light-headed or any type of pain.

Buddy system

As you get older, losing your balance and your confidence when trying new things is easy to do. Having a workout partner can help you gain back your confidence and boost your self-esteem by having someone else to share in your enthusiasm about your new workout experience and help you avoid injury by having someone else around. And did I mention that exercising is just a *lot* more fun when you do it in pairs? It's much easier to get motivated to go to the gym or simply leave the house and take a walk if you know someone is waiting and depending on you. So take your partner or pick a friend and use the buddy system when you exercise to help motivate you and keep you safe at the same time!

Core Routine to Help Maintain Balance

The following exercises are specifically designed to be accessible to anyone — even someone with physical limitations due to age or injury. None of these moves require you to get down on the ground or to assume complicated positions. These full-body exercises are simple and straightforward to help increase your range of motion, from your head to your toes.

Before you begin, remember these tips for keeping your balance:

- ✔ **Ask someone to exercise along with you or just watch you the first few times** (just in case you lose your balance).
- ✔ **Use a chair or table or couch or other piece of heavy furniture for balance.**
- ✔ **Once you're comfortable and steady, try using only one finger to hold on as you exercise.** When you feel comfortable with one fingertip, try the following exercises without holding anything. Build your confidence slowly and take your time . . . and most of all, have fun!

Hip extension

Starting with the hips and lower back, this core strengthener is a good exercise to help keep you balanced. You can use a chair or the back of a couch for assistance — just like ballet dancers do when they warm up at a ballet barre.

1. **Stand about a foot away from a chair and keep your feet slightly apart as you stand tall.**

2. **Bend forward at your hips until you're at a 45-degree angle as you hold onto the chair for balance** (as shown in Figure 18-1a).

3. **Slowly extend or raise one leg behind you without bending your knee.** Point your toe like a dancer and keep your upper body at a 45-degree angle with the floor. Don't bend any farther when you raise your leg (see Figure 18-1b).

   Hold your leg and upper-body position for one second.

4. **Slowly lower your leg before repeating on the other side.**

   Alternate your legs until you have done eight to ten repetitions on each side.

For the best results, when you do a hip extension:

- Keep your shoulder blades down and your upper body relaxed.

- Keep your back straight, not rounded.

- Keep your back gentle and slowly progress into a deeper stretch — don't bounce or force the stretch.

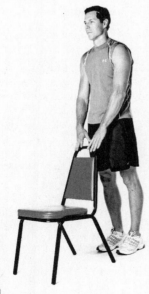 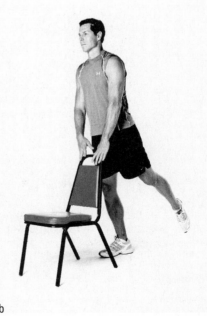

Figure 18-1: Hip extension.

a   b

Hip flexion

This exercise works the back, hips, and legs. It's simple and effective for strengthening your core. The rule is: Any time you lift your leg or foot off the ground; you call on your core muscles to keep you from falling.

Try this with or without holding onto something . . . depending on your individual level of fitness.

To do this exercise, follow these steps:

1. **Stand up tall and as straight as possible.** If you need to, hold onto a table or chair for balance (see Figure 18-2a).

2. **Slowly bend one knee up and toward your chest, without bending at your waist or hips.** Your arms should be in the airplane position out to your sides for balance (see Figure 18-2b).

   Once you become more advanced, you can place both hands on your hips.

3. **Hold your bent knee up for one second before slowly lowering your leg all the way down.**

4. **Repeat on the other leg.**

   Alternate legs until you've completed eight to ten repetitions on each leg.

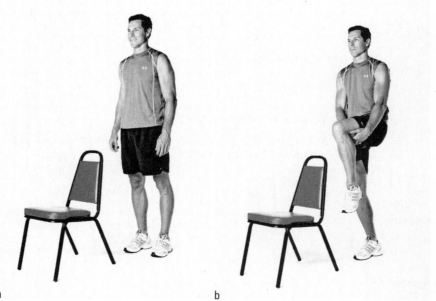

Figure 18-2:
Hip flexion.

a   b

The hip flexion exercise can be done effectively and safely as long as you:

✔ Keep your shoulders and hips facing forward and your knees slightly bent.

✔ Breathe through the exercise.

✔ Avoid holding the position if you feel tension or pain.

Side leg raises

Side leg raises work your lower back and hip muscles. Your legs will feel stronger from this core strengthener, too. You will need a chair or a heavy piece of furniture to hold onto for this exercise.

To do this exercise, follow these steps:

1. **Stand up straight, directly behind a chair for support with your feet slightly apart (see Figure 18-3a).**

2. **Slowly lift one leg out to the side about 8 to 12 inches.**

   Keep your back and both legs straight (as shown in Figure 18-3b).

   Keep your toes pointing forward during this exercise, and don't let your leg turn out.

3. **Slowly lower your leg back down to the ground before repeating with the other leg.**

   Alternate legs until you've completed eight to ten repetitions on each leg.

It's important that the chair is sturdy and stable (so don't pick one that's unbalanced or has wheels!).

When you do this exercise remember to:

✔ Keep your back straight at all times.

✔ Keep your butt squeezed and contracted — don't tuck your pelvis under while you're standing

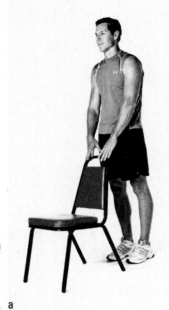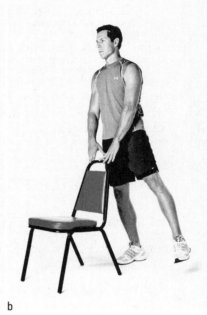

Figure 18-3:
Side leg
raises.

a   b

Standing core release

Using the back of a chair for support in the standing core release allows you to reach the waist (oblique muscles) and back muscles that are difficult to release without lying on the floor. You can feel the release in your back, abs, and even the top part of your hip.

To do this stretch, follow these steps:

1. **Stand with the back of your chair about a foot from your right side.**

2. **Place your right hand on the top of the back of the chair.**

3. **Stand with your feet about 12 inches or 1 foot apart, your knees slightly bent and your toes pointing forward (see Figure 18-4a).**

4. **Inhale and reach your left arm directly overhead with your palm facing inward.**

   Use the muscles in your upper back to keep your shoulder blade down. This should keep space between your shoulder and ear.

5. **As you exhale, lean to the right, keeping your right hand on the back of the chair for support and your hip and leg anchored to the floor (see Figure 18-4b).**

6. **Hold this stretch for 30 seconds or four to five slow, deep breaths.**

7. **Repeat on the other side.**

If you notice tension in your shoulders, instead of reaching with a straight arm, keep your elbow bent. The movement should come from your waist, and not your shoulder.

You get the most from the standing core release if you:

✔ **Keep your shoulders and hips facing forward and your knees slightly bent.**

✔ **Breathe through the stretch.**

✔ **Avoid holding the stretch if you feel tension or pain.**

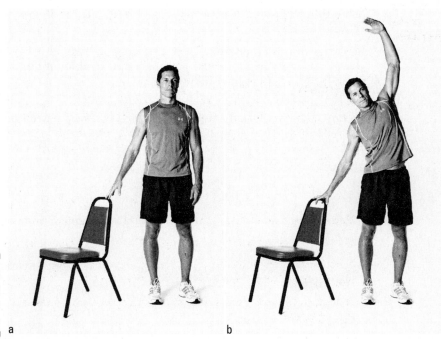

Figure 18-4:
Standing
core
release.

a   b

Seated Core Routine for Strong Abs

The next three exercises modify some very popular abdominal and core exercises, making them perfect for older adults. The sit-up is done in a chair along with the core and spinal twist. All of these exercises are fun and still very effective when done seated!

Seated sit-up

Doing seated sit-ups is a good way to work on your abdominals and lower back as well as your quadriceps, butt, and hamstrings without having to lie on the floor and do a sit-up! Actually, anyone can do this exercise; it's not just for seniors. It helps you strengthen your core and helps you get up and down from a seated position without losing your balance.

To do this exercise, follow these steps:

1. **Sit tall in a chair with your arms extended in front of you (see Figure 18-5a).**

2. **Tighten your abdominals before (pulling) pressing through with your heels as you straighten your legs and straighten up to a standing position (refer to Figure 18-5b).**

3. **Hold for a few seconds before sitting back down in the chair as you keep your core muscles tight and engaged to help you sit back down.**

    Repeat eight to ten times.

The seated sit-up works your body best when you:

- Keep your back straight and your shoulder blades down.
- Keep your knees pointing forward — don't let them flair out to the sides.

Seated core rotation

The biggest benefit to having strong lower-back muscles is that you're less prone to injury. Now that's good news for anyone, young or old. Both the seated core rotation and the seated core stretch (see "Seated core stretch," below) benefit the abdominal and back muscle groups.

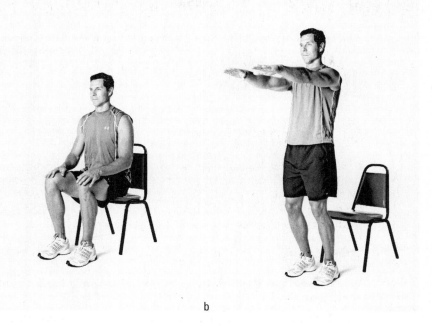

Figure 18-5:
Seated
sit-up.

a   b

With these two exercises you increase the flexibility in your spine, which in turn helps prevent injuries and makes everyday movements easier.

To do this stretch, follow these steps:

1. **Sit up tall on a sturdy chair with your feet flat on the floor and close together, knees at a right angle.**

2. **Anchor your right hand on the side of the chair as you place your left hand on the outside of your right thigh (see Figure 18-6a).**

3. **Inhale and, as you exhale, twist your torso to the right and look back over your shoulder (see Figure 18-6b).**

4. **Hold the stretch for about ten seconds.**

   Try to make a mental note of a stationary object you see that's about at eye level.

5. **Release and come back to center.**

6. **Inhale again, and as you exhale repeat on the opposite side.**

   Find the same object you were looking at, but this time try to find another object that's past it.

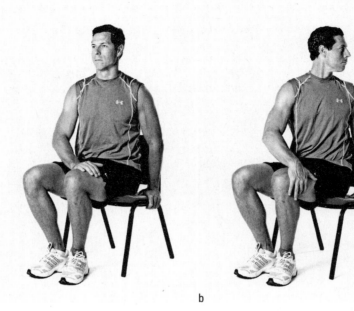

Figure 18-6:
Seated core
rotation.

a   b

For the seated core rotation, remember to:

✔ Keep your feet flat on the floor.

✔ Keep your knees and feet together and facing the front.

✔ Find an object that's at eye level — don't look down.

Seated core stretch

Tight chest muscles cause a lot of older adults to round their shoulders and hunch over. Increasing flexibility in the chest and upper body guarantees more freedom of movement as you age. Try this core exercise to help stretch out your chest and shoulders.

To do this stretch, follow these steps:

1. **Sit up tall on the front edge of a chair (see Figure 18-7a).**

2. **Reach behind your back with both arms and link your forearms (see Figure 18-7b).**

3. **Inhale and as you exhale, squeeze your shoulder blades together.**

4. **Hold the pose for about 30 seconds or four to five slow, deep breaths.**

5. **Repeat the same exercise with the other hand on top.**

If your range of motion is limited in your shoulders, and/or you feel pain or discomfort, try performing this core stretch one arm at a time. Instead of grabbing both elbows at the same time, reach only one arm across the midline of your back and with your other hand grab hold of your wrist or forearm.

Remember theses tips as you perform the seated core stretch:

✔ Keep your eyes looking forward.

✔ Maintain good posture throughout the stretch.

✔ Avoid allowing your back to arch when you squeeze your shoulder blades together.

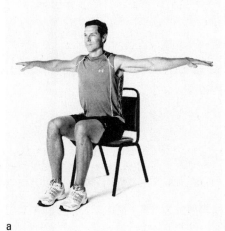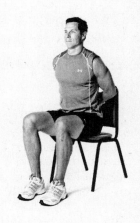

Figure 18-7:
Seated core stretch.

a

b

Should you exercise if you have arthritis?

The big question these days is, how much exercise should you do if you're diagnosed with arthritis? Generally, if you have a flare-up in a joint, that's the time to rest and let your medication do its job. As the inflammation decreases and the pain subsides, you can gradually return to exercise. The key word is *gradually*. If you experience pain, that's your cue to stop.

However, we've come a long way from the time when people believed that if they had arthritis they shouldn't exercise. Now we know that exercise is an important part of treating the disease. Why? Because, if you don't take care of the muscles that surround the joint, range of motion will be lost and stiffness and pain increase. The goal of people with arthritis should be to limit the progression of the existing damage in the affected joint or joints, which is most effectively accomplished by strengthening and stretching the muscles that surround the joints.

Arthritis is defined as inflammation of the joint or joints that is accompanied by swelling and pain which affects the spinal column, hips, ankles, and knee joints. Arthritis currently affects more than 40 million people, and within a year over a million more people will have it. Strength training alleviates arthritis symptoms and slows the aging process by building stronger muscles, bones, and connective tissue. The American Heart Association recommends that for muscular strength and endurance, sedentary adults need to use strength training at least twice per week. Although aerobic exercise is great for improving your overall cardiovascular system, it doesn't prevent your body from losing muscle tissue. To maintain muscle mass during seniorhood and to gain the relief you're looking for from arthritis pain, you must perform exercises with weights throughout the latter years of your life.

In addition to the arthritis information above, hip flexors, knees, and ankle joints can become stiff from being sedentary or leading an inactive lifestyle. Exercise can relieve this stiffness by promoting greater flexibility and mobility in your joints and throughout your entire body. Remember to always consult your doctor before starting any new exercise program.

Part VI
The Part of Tens

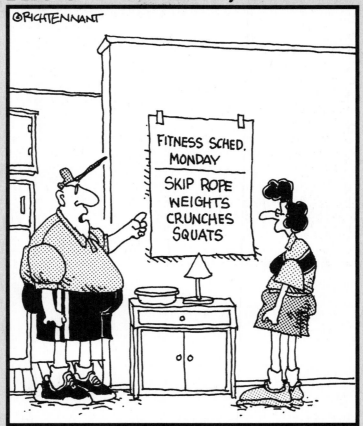

The 5th Wave   By Rich Tennant

FITNESS SCHED.
MONDAY

SKIP ROPE
WEIGHTS
CRUNCHES
SQUATS

"I AM following the schedule! Today I skipped the rope, then I skipped the weights, then I skipped the crunches."

In this part . . .

It is a hallowed tradition in the *For Dummies* series to end each book with a top-ten list, and in this book we end with three of them. In Chapter 19, I list ten best ways to train your core, and in Chapter 20, I show you ten core-conscious dietary changes you can make to trim your mid-section. In Chapter 21, I list ten lifestyle changes you can make to improve core strength. Finally, in Chapter 22, I show you ten of my favorite moves.

Chapter 19

Ten Best Ways to Train Your Core

A weak back is your body's way of telling you that your abs are weak. Your back and abs go hand in hand — together they make up your core. Think of core training as preventive medicine that creates balance between your back and abs, and returns your body to its natural, pain-free state.

This chapter gives you ten fast and fun ways to shore up your core. You can do the exercises outdoors or with a partner to make them more interesting and fun. Of course core training is only one tool in the battle against the bulge. You'll want to increase your cardio and head to Chapter 20 to see how diet and nutrition can really make a big difference.

Balance It

Here's an amazing exercise you can do with your exercise ball without even trying; you won't even break a sweat! Sit on your exercise ball instead of in your office chair for just one hour a day and you'll get tighter abs and a stronger back! Just by sitting up straight and sucking in your tummy, you improve your core strength and your balance at the same time. To keep from falling off the ball, you have to keep your feet flat on the floor and pull your abs in tight. Because the ball is round, you can't just plop yourself into it any old way like you can in a chair. See where I'm going with this? You're forced to strengthen your core.

Crunch It

One of the most effective methods for relieving belly fat and strengthening those abs is crunching them! Bringing your upper body to your lower body trains both the upper and lower parts of your abdominal muscles.

Here's an easy yet effective crunch: Grab an exercise ball and lie on the floor with your knees bent and feet flat on the floor. Place the ball between your ankles and bring your upper body to your lower body, or bring your knees to your elbows. This crunch works both your upper and lower abs and is much easier to do than a conventional ball sit-up.

For crunching it, I recommend the abs exercises I describe in the Chapter 6 for a killer core workout. These core exercises are very effective for targeting your core and will help you focus on the midsection of your body.

Fix It with Cardio

The best prevention against tummy fat is to stay low in body fat — and that means less belly fat. Doing 60 minutes of cardio exercise at least three times a week helps you maintain a low percentage of body fat, which in turn helps your six-pack peek through.

Jumping rope for 5 to 10 minutes at a time does the trick (ever see a boxer with belly fat?) and also helps keep your joints flexible. Or you can use a mini-trampoline like the Reebok Rebounder to do cardio that also helps train your abs and back. As you perform small bounces on the trampoline, your circulation increases to help flush out fatty deposits in your legs and your belly area.

Other great forms of cardio are running sprints, doing jumping jacks, or performing other activities that get your heart rate elevated and can be done consistently for at least 30 minutes. In fact, try to work in 30 minutes of cardio a day, five days a week if a full 60 minutes, three days a week just doesn't leave you enough time; you'll get the same results. Remember, consistency is the key!

Stretch It Out

Whether you lead a sedentary lifestyle or are an elite athlete, tight muscles in your abs, hips, back, and buttocks can put so much strain and stress on your lower back that the end result is low back pain. One solution that has been proven to be effective is regular stretching (see *Stretching For Dummies* by yours truly).

In this book, Chapter 14 gives you a ton of stretches for the core area (hips, abs, back, and butt), or if you're feeling tightness in your lower back try the routine I laid out in Chapter 18 that is specifically designed to help relieve low back tightness and may be for seniors but can help anyone! Never forget — a healthy core is a strong and flexible back.

Walk It Out

If you want to banish belly fat and strengthen your core, but rigorous exercise is the last activity you want to add to your routine, take a walk every night after dinner.

Walking is the best form of exercise for getting rid of belly fat and training your core (and you'll enjoy your neighborhood at the same time). When you take long strides, you work all the muscles that support your stomach, back, and pelvis. Plus walking is easy to do, and you only need to do it 30 minutes a day, five days a week. Trust me, it works better than skipping dessert (although that doesn't hurt)!

Cycle Through It

When you're cycling, you use your legs to spin the wheel and your abdominals and back muscles to push the pedals. Perfect for core training! Combining it with a few bicycle crunches (see Chapter 5) which helps target the same area by bringing your knees to your chest is a great way to work your core. In addition, you get the extra benefit of a cardio workout, which helps reduce belly fat.

A spinning class at a gym uses a stationary bike with a 40-pound wheel that allows you to increase and decrease the tension during the class. A spinning class burns more than 500 calories and takes biking to a whole new level. Try it; I know you'll like it!

Plank It

The plank exercise is one of the best core strengthening exercise and can be found in several chapters of this book (see Chapters 5, 11, and 12). The plank position requires you to pull in your abs while you stay lifted in a push-up position with your glutes squeezed together and your back straight.

The plank exercise energizes your entire body. It's used in all yoga sun salutations and other poses (see Chapter 12). It is also a Pilates-based exercise (see Chapter 11), which is used in many of Joseph Pilates's exercises to help strengthen the core of the body. So next time you're short on time, roll out of bed, drop down to the floor, and plank it!

Lengthen It

Any exercise that lengthens your core engages the muscles through stretching. In Chapters 11 and 12 of this book, the yoga and Pilates exercises use extending and lengthening exercises to help you achieve core definition.

Dancers always tend to look long and lean because they have great posture. They achieve this by having strong abdominal and back muscles. It all works hand in hand — strong abs, strong back, and good posture. It's all good!

Suck It In

In many cases, people just aren't in the habit of pulling in their tummies and sucking it in! To suck in your stomach, pretend you're tightening a belt around your waist as you're standing or sitting tall throughout the day. This technique gives you a visual reminder and helps you keep your stomach muscles tight and taut instead of letting them go slack!

Twist It

Twisting your core helps define your waist by working the *obliques* (muscles that run along the waist). The bicycle crunch I mentioned earlier (in Chapter 5) is very effective for working this area, and that's why I like it so much. Any exercise that twists your upper body requires strong abs and back muscles.

Sports that use a twisting motion include golf and baseball. In both of them, you have to twist to hit the ball. Both sports engage the core and help develop the kind of strength you need to be a good player. Think Tiger Woods!

Chapter 20

Ten Core-Conscious Dietary Changes You Can Easily Make

*E*xperts support the fact that calories (in excess) are what make you fat . . . duh! And because calories create the energy you need to get through your day, exercise is very important to burn them off. But just as in everything in life, moderation is the key! And the bottom line is, if you eat more calories than you burn off, you create an imbalance in your body and gain weight. It's that simple!

So what is the key to limiting calories or practicing portion control? And how do you find the right balance between the foods you eat and the amount of energy you burn on a daily basis? In this chapter, I talk about these and other ways you can take control of your diet by reducing fatty foods, cutting back on carbs, drinking lots of water, and eating more of the right things like salads, lean protein, less dairy, less salt- and sugar-laden foods, and a few other tips that will help get you started on the path to a healthier you.

Reduce Fatty Foods

Basically, fats come in two kinds: one healthy (in moderation, of course) and one not so healthy. And because I'm an optimist, let's start with the healthy fats.

Natural healthy fats, or "green light" fats, as I prefer to call them, are olive oil (my personal fave), nuts that are dry-roasted to preserve the healthy oils, avocado, and even canola oil. Interestingly, the body really can't distinguish between a Snickers bar and a handful of nuts when it comes to calories. But it does know the difference when it comes to the *nutritional* value in these two items and how the body breaks them down.

Now for the unhealthy man-made stuff: trans fats and saturated fats.

Trans fats are anything man-made, like vegetable oil, which most desserts and baked goods contain. The best way to confirm that a fat is not a healthy choice is to leave it sitting out on the counter and watch it harden!

Saturated fats are animal fats, which are found in red meat and butter (darn). When you hear that something is high in saturated fat, you know to limit it or steer clear of it altogether.

Your body does need fat to function properly, though, and for healthy skin and nails. So when you buy a salad dressing — or anything else, for that matter — that contains fat, go natural and choose olive oil and vinegar instead of ranch. And, yes, choose guacamole instead of spinach and artichoke dip, because you never know how much fat is added to that. Yikes!

Cut Back on Carbs

Carb-free diets? No way. Eating only protein? Now that's high in fat. As with fats, there are good carbs and bad carbs. And your body and your brain both need carbs to function properly. Without carbs, or carbohydrates, you would have no energy and would be listless.

Healthy carbs are anything made with whole grain: whole-grain pastas, rice, and, of course, breads. Now here's where portion control comes in: You really shouldn't eat more than two slices of whole-wheat bread or 1 cup of rice because it all adds up. Remember, we're focusing on calories and trying to add them to your diet in the healthiest way possible. So do your math and eat a sandwich, but certainly not at the same time as the rice, silly!

Eat Lean Protein

Gotta have the protein — just not too much of it, and it's gotta be lean. Lean proteins are white meats, like chicken and turkey. Fish is always a good choice, along with shellfish, for getting your daily protein. And if you choose salmon, tuna, or a few other types of fish that are off the beaten path (sardines, yuck!), you'll get your heart-healthy fats, better known as omega-3 fatty acids. You can also take omega-3 supplements in pill form, but I think it's always best to get it from your diet naturally.

Veal, pork (the other white meat), and beef are also good choices for lean proteins. But look for leaner cuts that have less than 5 percent fat (which means they're 95 percent lean cuts).

When it comes to serving size, I usually use the palm of my hand to measure portions, but since there are many different palm sizes out there, the rule of thumb (no pun intended) is 8 ounces or 1 cup of lean protein three times a day.

You can also choose veggie proteins, like beans and soy products. Both of these offerings taste fantastic and are very high in protein — plus they'll keep your core looking lean and mean!

Say Bye-Bye to Dairy

Bad cheese, good soy! Bad sour cream, good yogurt. Maybe I've been around kids too long, but I'm giving you the *CliffsNotes* version of my shopping list. And I love cheese! But all that great French brie adds up and is fattening, as you know by now from reading the previous segment on fats, because it hardens when you leave it sitting out on the counter (darn, again).

However, if you start reading labels and make some smart choices, like drinking 1 percent milk and eating plain yogurt or even no-sugar-added yogurt, you can keep some dairy in your diet and still get a healthy core. You just have to watch what they mix it with — usually fat or sugar. So do read those labels— and that's an order!

Drink Fewer Margaritas

Alcohol raises cortisol levels, which is a hormone responsible for storing fat. And the kind of fat that cortisol regulates is belly fat! So if you want to have a strong core, you don't want belly fat, right? You can still have a drink to celebrate a special occasion or just let loose once in a while, but you have to make smart choices.

Consider this funny story: My friend went to a Weight Watchers meeting and told me she spoke for the first time on the very last night of the sessions. She stood up and said, "If you're going to have a margarita, just skip the drink and have the shot of tequila instead!" Boy, is she right! The sugary high-caloric content of a margarita is astronomical, whereas a shot of 80-proof alcohol is only 1,000 calories. Now, of course, I'm not suggesting you use 200 calories on just alcohol, because you want to make smart choices for your core. Even better would be choosing a glass of wine, which is around 100 calories or a glass of beer, which is 150 calories. You may get to have only one, but I'll bet you'll enjoy it even more knowing that it must last you all night!

Just Say "No" to Sugary Soft Drinks

I find in a lot of hidden calories in people's diets in soda. And unless you're drinking Diet Coke or Diet Pepsi, you're getting a ton of sugar and a ton of calories (Paris Hilton says diet soda is for fat people . . . yikes!). I have a simple solution for that: Replace soda with water! Yep, water has no calories and it is good for your core. The more water you drink, the more toxins and bad stuff you flush out of your system, and the more weight you lose. Drinking water is my number one fitness tip for my clients when we start working together. And it's a lot cheaper than soda!

Try this fun tip at home (kids, leave this to your mom and dad): Try drinking your weight in ounces of water throughout the day. So let's say you weigh 120 pounds — you would want to drink 120 ounces of water from the time you wake up until the time you go to bed. You'll feel less sluggish, save lots of money not buying soda, and spend lots of time going to the bathroom. Those three things I can guarantee because I've been there, done that! And it works.

Eat More Salads

I remember hearing Shaquille O'Neal say when someone asked him how he lost all his weight, "I ate a lot of salad." I'll bet he did, that big guy! But I'll also bet he didn't use much salad dressing, because that's where all the hidden calories come from.

Salad is always a good option when you're trying to trim your core. However, what you put on it can really make a difference. Some low-calorie offerings are pretty good these days, but it's best to stick with lemon or vinegar with olive oil. Creamy dressings are always packed with fat and calories, which might make you eat more salad but cancels out the good you're trying to accomplish by filling up with roughage.

Try adding dried legumes or beans, adding tuna with some garbanzo beans, or topping your salad with beets and carrots for some healthy options. Just be sure to skip the dressing, or you'll look like Shaq — just not as tall!

Don't Eat after 7 p.m.

You've probably heard that eating late helps pack on the pounds. If you're eating every three to four hours throughout the day, as you should be, plus adding two to three snacks, you won't be hungry later in the day anyway. If you do eat at night, you go to sleep on a full stomach, which slows your metabolism significantly and keeps you from getting a good night's rest.

Breakfast is exactly what it's named for: break the fast! Not eating after 7 p.m. and waiting until you wake up in the morning gives your body a chance to rest and rejuvenate so you wake up bright-eyed and bushy-tailed. That's where the principle of eating a good breakfast comes in. If you don't start your engine with something good in the morning, you're running on empty all day and you aren't giving your body the rest it needs. So start the day out right with a good, hot breakfast. Follow that with two more meals and three snacks, and you'll be trimming your core all day long.

Snack on Fewer Salty Foods and More Fat-Free Pudding

Salt equals water retention, making you look puffy and doing nothing for your core except making you look bloated. And everything contains salt these days — especially many fat-free foods. How do you think they make these foods taste so good? They replace all that fat with two ingredients: salt and water. Have you ever tried cooking with low-fat margarine? When the pan heats up, the water runs to one side of the pan while the "fat" pools in the middle. Well, that's the secret to many fat-free foods — extra salt for taste and extra water to dilute the fat. Now instead of doing something good for yourself, you're actually consuming extra sodium and calories that you don't have to.

Snacking on fat-free chocolate pudding instead of salty chips, and eating microwave popcorn (without extra butter) are healthier choices you can make for your core. No hidden calories there — and no bloating!

Drink Lots of H$_2$O

As I mentioned earlier in reference to sugary soft drinks, water is the answer for flushing out the toxins and extra fluids your body is holding on to. It seems strange, but the more water you drink, the less your body retains.

Consider these guidelines for drinking water daily:

✔ Drink 80 ounces (eight glasses) of water daily. Drinking water enlarges the cells in your body, so it makes you feel full! Because you're less hungry, you eat less.

✔ Drinking a glass of water before or along with meals is another good option to fill you up.

✔ Water reduces muscle soreness by helping to flush out the lactic acid that builds up in your muscles from strenuous exercise. Drinking water helps replenish the water content in your body and serves as a checks-and-balances system to make sure everything is operating smoothly. You'll be taking a lot more trips to the bathroom, but at least you'll be going!

Jumping rope flushes out water!

Jumping rope for ten minutes three times a week is one of the most effective ways to improve cardiovascular fitness and reduce cellulite. In one of my other books, *Lose That Baby Fat* (M. Evans and Company, Inc.), I mention that one study suggests that you can improve overall physical fitness in as little as five minutes a day.

Women especially will appreciate of the benefits of jumping rope because it reduces cellulite and creates more shapely calves. Tired and weak joints get a boost as well. Fifteen minutes spent jumping rope translate into 200 fewer calories to worry about, which is the equivalent number lost on a 30-minute run. Plus, when done properly, skipping rope is kinder to your knees and hips than running.

Chapter 21

Ten Household Items You Can Use to Help Improve Core Strength

In This Chapter

▶ Being spontaneous with your core exercises

▶ Exercising with everyday items

You already know exercise is important, but it's also extremely helpful to do a little bit each day. Why? Because frequent exercise, even in small amounts, provides several crucial benefits:

✔ **Maintains your fitness level:** Even when you're short on time or you missed your workout, performing calisthenics or a few simple exercises throughout the day helps maintain your fitness level that you've worked so hard to achieve.

✔ **Energizes you:** When you need an energy boost and there's no coffee or chocolate in sight, try a jumping jack or two to get oxygen to your brain. You'll feel great, and you'll skip the calories!

✔ **Relieves minor aches and pains:** Exercise relieves the stress created by inactivity or repetitive motions by increasing your circulation and keeping oxygen flowing to sore muscles.

So any time can be the right time to exercise when you're at home. And believe it or not, your home is full of core-strengthening aids. The rest of the chapter points out common items you can use in your fitness routine. Now you *really* have no excuse not to stretch!

A Chair from Your Kitchen

Sitting in a chair too long and too often doesn't loosen and relax your muscles; it actually shortens certain muscles, such as your hamstrings, hip flexors, and calves. Nevertheless, a chair can be a very useful and effective prop for exercising. And I bet you have a chair in just about every room of the house.

In Chapter 18, you'll see a series of exercises that can be done with a chair including the seated sit-up. To do this exercise, sit in a chair and extend your arms out in front of you. Now rise to a standing position. Notice how you're forced to use your core. Pause for a moment before sitting back down in the chair. Repeat 10 to 15 times.

Be careful, especially at work, that you don't use a chair with wheels. You can use any type of chair, as long as it's sturdy and stable.

A Beam or Rafter in Your House

Just like in the movie *Rocky,* you can hang from an open beam in your house or garage to do a pull-up. At first you'll probably only be able to hold yourself up for a few seconds, but as your grip gets stronger, you'll be able to chin-up or pull yourself up to really feel the strength in your core increasing.

If you're having trouble with this exercise, put a chair underneath the beam to help you reach it and grab on.

Your Coffee Table in the Living Room

Although you may think of your coffee table as being a good place to rest your coffee, this versatile piece of furniture makes for a great piece of exercise equipment:

- ✔ It's strong and usually made of wood, so you can do dips off of it without being afraid that it will break under your weight.
- ✔ It's off the floor, which makes it easier to get into a lot of different positions.
- ✔ It's in hotel rooms, so even when you travel, you can get a core workout!

Try some of the exercises as shown in Chapter 13 using your coffee table. It's a great way to work your core.

Your Desk in Your Home Office

Your desk at home can be an excellent prop for exercising. When you need to take a break from sitting in front of the computer, you don't have to go very far to move some different muscles. Here's how to do deep lunges, using your desk for support:

1. Stand in front of your desk and place both hands on top, making sure you're an arm's length away from it.

2. Lean forward into a lunge position so your right knee bends and your left leg is extended behind you.

3. Drop your left knee slowly to the floor as you tighten your stomach muscles to hold your body weight stable.

4. Inhale deeply as you press back up to a standing position, using your abs and back to keep you standing tall.

5. Repeat the core strengthener with the left leg.

If you don't have a desk handy, you can do this exercise using your dining room table or a hip-high windowsill.

A Doorway in Your Bathroom

A doorway is a great exercise prop because it's both stable and large enough to have many different applications.

Try this shoulder stretch using a doorjamb:

1. Grab onto the molding over the top of the door with your fingertips.

2. Bend your knees slightly, but keep your feet on the floor until you feel a stretch in your abdominals and back muscles.

3. Grab onto the sides of the doorway and bend forward as if you were going to touch your toes.

If you're not tall enough to reach the top of the door, you can use a stepstool.

Water Jugs in Your Kitchen

Okay, now I know I'm a total nerd because I find myself doing this all the time when I refill the water machine. But those 1- to 2-gallon jugs with the handles make for a good piece of resistance equipment, don't they?

You can curl (and press, if you're really feeling energetic) your water jugs (or old milk jugs filled with water) to give your biceps a workout, as well as tone your core as you transition the movement through it. Adding weight to your core allows you to tighten this area while you maintain proper posture and focus on the individual muscles you're working (see Chapter 10 for adding weights to your core).

A Towel in Your Bathroom

For core stretching, nothing beats a good, old-fashioned bath towel or smaller hand towel to help you achieve the stretch. It doesn't matter whether you're attempting a stretch for the upper or the lower body; using a towel to increase your reach makes the stretch more comfortable. See Chapter 14 for a few examples of stretches you can do with a towel.

The Steps in Your House

Every time you walk up and down the steps, guess what you're working? Yep, your butt — but also your abs, hips, back, and core! I live in a three-story home, and I'm convinced I don't have to do anything else but walk up and down the stairs about 50 times a day to stay fit. Now try carrying laundry and kids up and down, too, and you'll see what I mean. If you have stairs in your house, use them! When you're done, stretch out your feet and legs with the following exercise:

1. **Stand on the bottom step with only the ball of your right foot pressed down as your left foot remains beside it. Inhale deeply.**

   Make sure you hold on to a railing or something stable to prevent you from falling.

2. **As you exhale, slowly lower your heel until you feel a comfortable stretch in your calf.**

3. **Hold the stretch for 10 to 15 seconds.**

4. **Try to gently drop your heel a little lower until you feel a deeper stretch in your calf.**

5. **Repeat the stretch on your other leg.**

An excellent variation to help you stretch your calf more deeply is to slightly bend the knee of the leg you're stretching. You should feel a difference at the base of your calf.

A Wall in Your House

You can use a wall to support any stretch. It's smooth and wide and (I know this sounds a little obvious) adjacent to the floor. It's precisely because a wall is adjacent to the floor that you have two firm, stable sources of support.

You can do push-ups (see Chapter 13) using the wall instead of your coffee table. The exercise is easier when you use the wall, but it's just as effective at toning your core, and it's especially good for strengthening your back.

When you're done with your push-up, turn around and put your back flat against the wall and bend forward from your hips to let your head and arms and everything else hang out. If you can't place your palms on the floor as in Chapter 13 (and face it, not many of us can), rest your hands on your shins for support. This is a great back and core strengthener.

A Book Lying on Your Nightstand

Sit on a big book to lift your hips off the floor just enough to take away some of the stress and strain of a tight lower back. When you don't feel that strain anymore, you can stretch forward to grasp your toes and focus on pulling your belly button to your spine without rounding your back.

Chapter 22

Ten Favorite Moves

This chapter is what I like to call a round-up chapter because I've pulled ten fast and fun exercises from this book to help shore up your core. Because these aren't new moves you can also try them out in the other workouts where they appear in this book.

Of course, core training is only one tool in the battle against the bulge. To really get ahead of the game, you need to increase your cardio and try some of the tips in Chapter 20 on how eating better can help speed up your goal to shrink your midsection.

Back Extensions

The back extension exercise seems simple, yet it is a powerful and effective back strengthener. It also targets the lower back, so if you have lower back problems, you may want to skip this exercise.

To do this exercise, follow these steps:

1. **Using a mat or towel, lie on your stomach and place your arms at your sides, with the palms facing up (see Figure 22-1a).**

2. **Pulling in or contracting your abdominal muscles, lift your chest a few inches off the floor, keeping your gaze straight ahead at all times (see Figure 22-1b).**

3. **Hold for a few seconds before lowering your chest back toward the ground.**

4. **Repeat this exercise three to five times and increase reps as exercise becomes easier.**

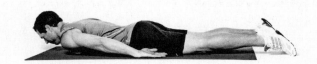

a

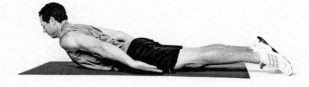

Figure 22-1:
Back
extensions.

b

Make sure you

- ✔ Tighten your butt or glutes to protect your lower back as you lift your chest off the floor.

- ✔ Tighten your abdominals throughout this move.

- ✔ Avoid lifting too high off the floor. Lift only to the point that you are not straining your back.

Plank

The plank is another top core exercise that targets the abdominals and back muscles. Stay strong and lifted during this exercise, and maintain a long, straight back.

To do this exercise, follow these steps:

1. **Lie face down, resting your forearms flat on the floor, and keep your elbows directly below your shoulders (see Figure 22-2a).**

   Your feet should be touching or no more than an inch apart.

2. **Lift your body off the floor using your forearms and toes, keeping your body as straight as possible. Maintain this position for as long as possible, and challenge yourself as you build up to longer periods in the plank position (see Figure 22-2b).**

3. **Hold the position for 10 to 15 seconds in the beginning or as long as you can before working your way up to holding the plank position for longer periods of time.**

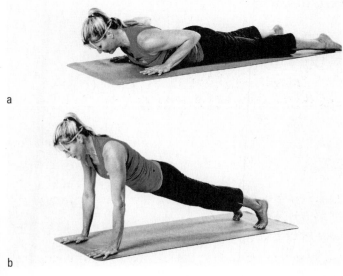

a

b

Figure 22-2:
Plank.

You don't want to forget these tips:

✔ Keep your back long and straight.

✔ Don't let your hips or knees drop toward the floor.

✔ Breathe steady and engage your abs.

Abdominal Crunch

Doing abdominal crunches not only works the abs but also strengthens the back and hips.

Make sure you keep your lower back in neutral spine when doing crunches to maintain proper form and support your lower back. If you let your lower back arch off the ground, you could strain it and pull a muscle. Not good!

To do this exercise, follow these steps:

1. **Lying on the floor, bend your knees and rest your feet flat on the floor (see Figure 22-3a).**

2. **As you tighten your abdominals and with your hands on either side of your head, slowly lift your shoulders from the floor toward your knees (see Figure 22-3b).**

3. **Hold the lift for a few seconds, and then slowly roll your shoulders back to the floor.**

   Complete ten repetitions.

While doing the ab crunch, remember to:

✔ Relax your neck as you curl up into a crunch.

✔ Keep your chin toward the ceiling and don't use your hands to pull your head off the floor.

✔ Maintain your neutral spine by pressing your lower back into the floor.

✔ Exhale as you curl up into the crunch and inhale as you release back down.

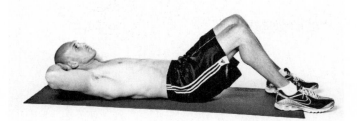

a

Figure 22-3:
Abdominal
crunch.

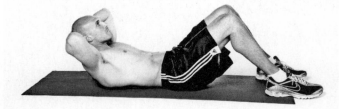

b

Double Crunch

This exercise tightens the lower abs and upper abs by bringing the upper and lower body together like an accordion. Be sure to return to starting position each time you finish the double crunch to help you get the best toning in your midsection possible.

To do this exercise, follow these steps:

1. **Keeping your knees bent and your feet off the floor, engage your abdominal muscles by pulling your belly button in toward your spine (see Figure 22-4a). Place your fingertips behind your head for support.**

2. **Pull your knees toward your chest, focusing on your abdominals as you bring your elbows toward your knees (see Figure 22-4b).**

3. **Slowly lower legs and arms back down to the starting position to complete one rep.**

   Aim for three sets of ten repetitions.

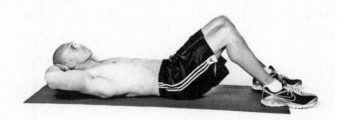

a

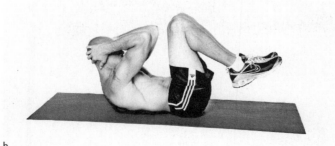

Figure 22-4:
Double
crunch.

b

Although it sounds more like your favorite ice cream rather than your favorite exercise, you can help burn off those double-crunch calories if you remember to:

✔ Hold the movement at the top before slowly letting your knees back down toward the floor

✔ Use your core muscles to control the movement.

✔ Let your head rest in your hands for support during the crunch. Don't pull on your head with your hands.

Oblique Crunches

The oblique crunch or side-lying crunch is a great addition to your core program because it targets the side muscles or obliques, helping whittle the waist.

To do this exercise, follow these steps:

1. **Lying on the floor or on a mat, bend your knees and clasp your hands behind your neck (see Figure 22-5a).**

2. **Lifting your upper torso, raise yourself slightly off the floor using your waist muscles or obliques (as shown in Figure 22-5b).**

   Bring your elbow toward your feet to target the waist.

3. **Return back down to the floor and repeat on other side after ten repetitions.**

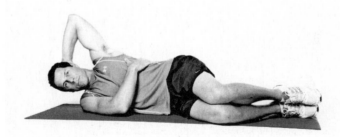

a

Figure 22-5: Oblique crunches or side-lying crunch.

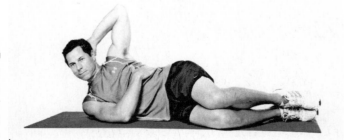

b

For these crunches, you need to be sure to:

✔ Engage your core throughout this entire exercise.

✔ Keep your knees on the ground and use your upper body to do the move.

✔ Avoid pulling on your head with your hands or it will strain your neck.

✔ Breathe!

Half-Up Twists

Half-up twists are great for the entire core and not just the abs. The back, butt, waist, and abdominals all get targeted with this challenging exercise.

To do this exercise, follow these steps:

1. **Sit up tall on the floor on a mat and put your hands on top of your knees.**

2. **Lean back until your arms are straight. Cross your arms in front of your chest with each hand holding an elbow (see Figure 22-6a).**

3. **Twist at the waist from side to side engaging your core as you sit up tall (as shown in Figure 22-6b).**

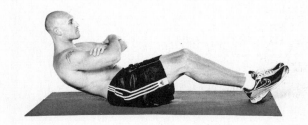

a

Figure 22-6:
Half-up twists — twisting at waist from side to side.

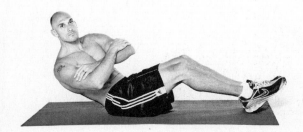

b

Here's what you need to remember while doing this exercise:

- ✔ Let your head follow the movement from side to side with you.

- ✔ Lean back and use the strength of your back to help you with this exercise.

- ✔ Sit up nice and tall. Don't let your shoulders and back round over.

Bicycle Crunches

This is the best exercise to work your rectus abdominus or ab muscle that runs right down the middle of your torso. The twisting and pulling motion you do with your knees and upper body is perfect for getting your core in shape fast and helps reduce your waist size too by working the obliques.

To do this exercise, follow these steps:

1. **Lie on your back with your knees bent and thighs perpendicular to the floor. Place your fingers just behind your ears (see Figure 22-7a).**

2. **Lift your shoulders off the floor as you straighten the right leg and bring the left knee in toward your right armpit.**

3. **Without relaxing the torso or returning your shoulders to the floor, repeat on the other side by straightening the left leg and pulling the right knee in toward the left armpit (as shown in Figure 22-7b).**

4. **Alternate the legs in a slow bicycling movement ten times on each side.**

Remember to bike your way to great abs with the following tips:

- ✔ Pull your abdominal muscles in for support.

- ✔ Allow your hips to drop down toward the ground — don't arch you back.

- ✔ Keep your breathing steady and strong — don't hold your breath.

- ✔ Avoid pulling you head with your hands to avoid straining your neck.

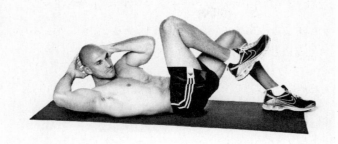

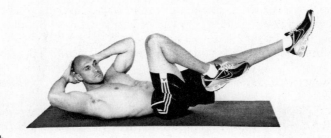

Figure 22-7:
Bicycle for
strong abs.

Reverse Crunches

By bringing your lower body to your upper body, you target your lower abs
and will see a tightening in this area faster than with other ab exercises.

To do this exercise, follow these steps:

1. **Keeping your knees bent and your feet off the floor, engage your
   abdominal muscles by pulling your belly button in toward your spine
   (see Figure 22-8a).**

2. **Pull your knees toward your chest, focusing on your abdominals as
   you keep your arms flat on the floor with palms facing down beside
   you (see Figure 22-8b).**

3. **Slowly lower hips and legs back down to the starting position to complete one rep.**

   Aim for one set of ten repetitions.

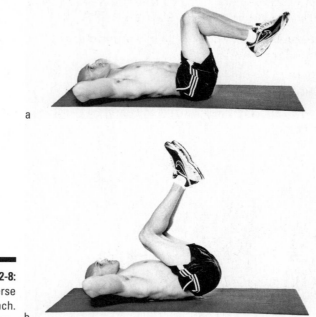

Figure 22-8:
Reverse
crunch.

Keep these tips in mind while doing a reverse crunch:

✔ Hold the movement at the top before slowly letting your knees back
down toward the floor

✔ Keep the pace slow and steady so you are using your core muscles to
control the movement — don't go too fast.

Plank Leg Lifts

Performing the plank with leg lifts makes for a killer core exercise. This exercise targets the abdominals and back while helping you maintain a straight,
healthy spine. Be sure to stay lifted and maintain a straight back during this
exercise. Great core strengthener. . . .

To do this exercise, follow these steps:

1. **Lie face down, resting your forearms flat on the floor; keep your
elbows directly below your shoulders.**

Your feet should be touching or no more than an inch apart.

2. **Lift your body off the floor using your forearms and toes, keeping your body as straight as possible (see Figure 22-9a).**

3. **Lift each leg one at a time off the floor before returning to the starting position (see Figure 22-9b).**

   You don't have to lift the legs more than half an inch to get the benefit of this exercise.

4. **Repeat for ten repetitions and increase repetitions when you feel comfortable.**

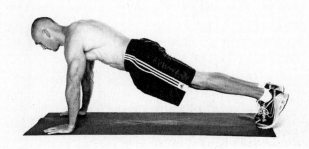

a

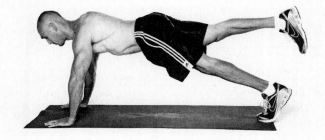

Figure 22-9:
Plank leg
lifts.

b

Maximize the benefits of this exercise by doing the following:

✔ Keep your back long and straight, in line from your head to your heels.

✔ Avoid letting your butt or hips drop toward the floor.

✔ Breathe steadily.

✔ Engage your abs and be sure to keep your leg straight and your butt contracted to help lift the leg.

Superman — Opposite Arm and Leg Extension

The Superman trains your entire core to work together properly, to provide stability and balance, while at the same time strengthening your abdominals. Remember, keeping your back strong and flexible is the best prevention against low back problems.

To do this stretch, follow these steps:

1. **Lie face down on a mat or the floor, with your arms extended overhead and palms facing down (as shown in Figure 22-10a).**

2. **At the same time, extend your right arm and your left leg out straight from your body and hold them out about three to five inches off the floor (see Figure 22-10b).**

   Imagine that strings are attached to your hand and foot, and that the strings are gently pulling your arm and leg away from each other, not up. You want to get the lengthening in your abdominal muscles and your spine, not shortening or compressing it.

3. **Hold the position for five to eight seconds, breathing comfortably and normally.**

4. **Lower your arm and leg, and return to the floor.**

5. **Repeat the exercise five or six more times on each side and increase repetitions when you feel comfortable.**

Make your Superman soar to new heights by remembering to:

✔ Keep your abdominals tight. Lax abdominals may place undue stress on your lower-back muscles.

✔ Not arch your back.

✔ Not lift your foot or hand higher than 3 to 5 inches off the floor.

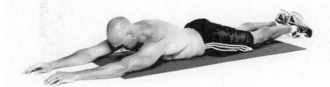

a

Figure 22-10:
Lifting your
opposite
arm and
leg in the
Superman
pose.

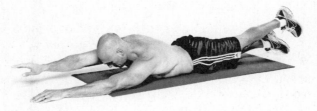

b

Index

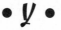

BUSINESS, CAREERS & PERSONAL FINANCE

Accounting For Dummies, 4th Edition*
978-0-470-24600-9

Bookkeeping Workbook For Dummies†
978-0-470-16983-4

Commodities For Dummies
978-0-470-04928-0

Doing Business in China For Dummies
978-0-470-04929-7

E-Mail Marketing For Dummies
978-0-470-19087-6

Job Interviews For Dummies, 3rd Edition*†
978-0-470-17748-8

Personal Finance Workbook For Dummies*†
978-0-470-09933-9

Real Estate License Exams For Dummies
978-0-7645-7623-2

Six Sigma For Dummies
978-0-7645-6798-8

Small Business Kit For Dummies, 2nd Edition*†
978-0-7645-5984-6

Telephone Sales For Dummies
978-0-470-16836-3

BUSINESS PRODUCTIVITY & MICROSOFT OFFICE

Access 2007 For Dummies
978-0-470-03649-5

Excel 2007 For Dummies
978-0-470-03737-9

Office 2007 For Dummies
978-0-470-00923-9

Outlook 2007 For Dummies
978-0-470-03830-7

PowerPoint 2007 For Dummies
978-0-470-04059-1

Project 2007 For Dummies
978-0-470-03651-8

QuickBooks 2008 For Dummies
978-0-470-18470-7

Quicken 2008 For Dummies
978-0-470-17473-9

Salesforce.com For Dummies, 2nd Edition
978-0-470-04893-1

Word 2007 For Dummies
978-0-470-03658-7

EDUCATION, HISTORY, REFERENCE & TEST PREPARATION

African American History For Dummies
978-0-7645-5469-8

Algebra For Dummies
978-0-7645-5325-7

Algebra Workbook For Dummies
978-0-7645-8467-1

Art History For Dummies
978-0-470-09910-0

ASVAB For Dummies, 2nd Edition
978-0-470-10671-6

British Military History For Dummies
978-0-470-03213-8

Calculus For Dummies
978-0-7645-2498-1

Canadian History For Dummies, 2nd Edition
978-0-470-83656-9

Geometry Workbook For Dummies
978-0-471-79940-5

The SAT I For Dummies, 6th Edition
978-0-7645-7193-0

Series 7 Exam For Dummies
978-0-470-09932-2

World History For Dummies
978-0-7645-5242-7

FOOD, GARDEN, HOBBIES & HOME

Bridge For Dummies, 2nd Edition
978-0-471-92426-5

Coin Collecting For Dummies, 2nd Edition
978-0-470-22275-1

Cooking Basics For Dummies, 3rd Edition
978-0-7645-7206-7

Drawing For Dummies
978-0-7645-5476-6

Etiquette For Dummies, 2nd Edition
978-0-470-10672-3

Gardening Basics For Dummies*†
978-0-470-03749-2

Knitting Patterns For Dummies
978-0-470-04556-5

Living Gluten-Free For Dummies†
978-0-471-77383-2

Painting Do-It-Yourself For Dummies
978-0-470-17533-0

HEALTH, SELF HELP, PARENTING & PETS

Anger Management For Dummies
978-0-470-03715-7

Anxiety & Depression Workbook For Dummies
978-0-7645-9793-0

Dieting For Dummies, 2nd Edition
978-0-7645-4149-0

Dog Training For Dummies, 2nd Edition
978-0-7645-8418-3

Horseback Riding For Dummies
978-0-470-09719-9

Infertility For Dummies†
978-0-470-11518-3

Meditation For Dummies with CD-ROM, 2nd Edition
978-0-471-77774-8

Post-Traumatic Stress Disorder For Dummies
978-0-470-04922-8

Puppies For Dummies, 2nd Edition
978-0-470-03717-1

Thyroid For Dummies, 2nd Edition†
978-0-471-78755-6

Type 1 Diabetes For Dummies*†
978-0-470-17811-9

---

* Separate Canadian edition also available
† Separate U.K. edition also available

Available wherever books are sold. For more information or to order direct: U.S. customers visit www.dummies.com or call 1-877-762-2974.
U.K. customers visit www.wileyeurope.com or call (0)1243 843291. Canadian customers visit www.wiley.ca or call 1-800-567-4797.

 WILEY

INTERNET & DIGITAL MEDIA

AdWords For Dummies
978-0-470-15252-2

Blogging For Dummies, 2nd Edition
978-0-470-23017-6

**Digital Photography All-in-One
Desk Reference For Dummies, 3rd Edition**
978-0-470-03743-0

Digital Photography For Dummies, 5th Edition
978-0-7645-9802-9

**Digital SLR Cameras & Photography
For Dummies, 2nd Edition**
978-0-470-14927-0

**eBay Business All-in-One Desk Reference
For Dummies**
978-0-7645-8438-1

eBay For Dummies, 5th Edition*
978-0-470-04529-9

eBay Listings That Sell For Dummies
978-0-471-78912-3

Facebook For Dummies
978-0-470-26273-3

The Internet For Dummies, 11th Edition
978-0-470-12174-0

Investing Online For Dummies, 5th Edition
978-0-7645-8456-5

iPod & iTunes For Dummies, 5th Edition
978-0-470-17474-6

MySpace For Dummies
978-0-470-09529-4

Podcasting For Dummies
978-0-471-74898-4

**Search Engine Optimization
For Dummies, 2nd Edition**
978-0-471-97998-2

Second Life For Dummies
978-0-470-18025-9

**Starting an eBay Business For Dummies
3rd Edition†**
978-0-470-14924-9

GRAPHICS, DESIGN & WEB DEVELOPMENT

**Adobe Creative Suite 3 Design Premium
All-in-One Desk Reference For Dummies**
978-0-470-11724-8

**Adobe Web Suite CS3 All-in-One Desk
Reference For Dummies**
978-0-470-12099-6

AutoCAD 2008 For Dummies
978-0-470-11650-0

**Building a Web Site For Dummies,
3rd Edition**
978-0-470-14928-7

**Creating Web Pages All-in-One Desk
Reference For Dummies, 3rd Edition**
978-0-470-09629-1

**Creating Web Pages For Dummies,
8th Edition**
978-0-470-08030-6

Dreamweaver CS3 For Dummies
978-0-470-11490-2

Flash CS3 For Dummies
978-0-470-12100-9

Google SketchUp For Dummies
978-0-470-13744-4

InDesign CS3 For Dummies
978-0-470-11865-8

**Photoshop CS3 All-in-One
Desk Reference For Dummies**
978-0-470-11195-6

Photoshop CS3 For Dummies
978-0-470-11193-2

Photoshop Elements 5 For Dummies
978-0-470-09810-3

SolidWorks For Dummies
978-0-7645-9555-4

Visio 2007 For Dummies
978-0-470-08983-5

Web Design For Dummies, 2nd Edition
978-0-471-78117-2

Web Sites Do-It-Yourself For Dummies
978-0-470-16903-2

Web Stores Do-It-Yourself For Dummies
978-0-470-17443-2

LANGUAGES, RELIGION & SPIRITUALITY

Arabic For Dummies
978-0-471-77270-5

Chinese For Dummies, Audio Set
978-0-470-12766-7

French For Dummies
978-0-7645-5193-2

German For Dummies
978-0-7645-5195-6

Hebrew For Dummies
978-0-7645-5489-6

Ingles Para Dummies
978-0-7645-5427-8

Italian For Dummies, Audio Set
978-0-470-09586-7

Italian Verbs For Dummies
978-0-471-77389-4

Japanese For Dummies
978-0-7645-5429-2

Latin For Dummies
978-0-7645-5431-5

Portuguese For Dummies
978-0-471-78738-9

Russian For Dummies
978-0-471-78001-4

Spanish Phrases For Dummies
978-0-7645-7204-3

Spanish For Dummies
978-0-7645-5194-9

Spanish For Dummies, Audio Set
978-0-470-09585-0

The Bible For Dummies
978-0-7645-5296-0

Catholicism For Dummies
978-0-7645-5391-2

The Historical Jesus For Dummies
978-0-470-16785-4

Islam For Dummies
978-0-7645-5503-9

**Spirituality For Dummies,
2nd Edition**
978-0-470-19142-2

NETWORKING AND PROGRAMMING

ASP.NET 3.5 For Dummies
978-0-470-19592-5

C# 2008 For Dummies
978-0-470-19109-5

Hacking For Dummies, 2nd Edition
978-0-470-05235-8

Home Networking For Dummies, 4th Edition
978-0-470-11806-1

Java For Dummies, 4th Edition
978-0-470-08716-9

**Microsoft® SQL Server™ 2008 All-in-One
Desk Reference For Dummies**
978-0-470-17954-3

**Networking All-in-One Desk Reference
For Dummies, 2nd Edition**
978-0-7645-9939-2

**Networking For Dummies,
8th Edition**
978-0-470-05620-2

SharePoint 2007 For Dummies
978-0-470-09941-4

**Wireless Home Networking
For Dummies, 2nd Edition**
978-0-471-74940-0

OPERATING SYSTEMS & COMPUTER BASICS

Mac For Dummies, 5th Edition
978-0-7645-8458-9

Laptops For Dummies, 2nd Edition
978-0-470-05432-1

Linux For Dummies, 8th Edition
978-0-470-11649-4

MacBook For Dummies
978-0-470-04859-7

**Mac OS X Leopard All-in-One
Desk Reference For Dummies**
978-0-470-05434-5

Mac OS X Leopard For Dummies
978-0-470-05433-8

Macs For Dummies, 9th Edition
978-0-470-04849-8

PCs For Dummies, 11th Edition
978-0-470-13728-4

Windows® Home Server For Dummies
978-0-470-18592-6

Windows Server 2008 For Dummies
978-0-470-18043-3

**Windows Vista All-in-One
Desk Reference For Dummies**
978-0-471-74941-7

Windows Vista For Dummies
978-0-471-75421-3

Windows Vista Security For Dummies
978-0-470-11805-4

SPORTS, FITNESS & MUSIC

Coaching Hockey For Dummies
978-0-470-83685-9

Coaching Soccer For Dummies
978-0-471-77381-8

Fitness For Dummies, 3rd Edition
978-0-7645-7851-9

Football For Dummies, 3rd Edition
978-0-470-12536-6

GarageBand For Dummies
978-0-7645-7323-1

Golf For Dummies, 3rd Edition
978-0-471-76871-5

Guitar For Dummies, 2nd Edition
978-0-7645-9904-0

**Home Recording For Musicians
For Dummies, 2nd Edition**
978-0-7645-8884-6

**iPod & iTunes For Dummies,
5th Edition**
978-0-470-17474-6

Music Theory For Dummies
978-0-7645-7838-0

Stretching For Dummies
978-0-470-06741-3

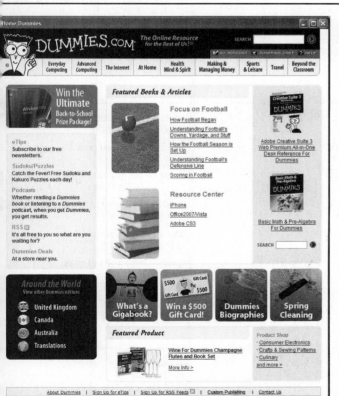

Get smart @ dummies.com®

- **Find a full list of Dummies titles**
- **Look into loads of FREE on-site articles**
- **Sign up for FREE eTips e-mailed to you weekly**
- **See what other products carry the Dummies name**
- **Shop directly from the Dummies bookstore**
- **Enter to win new prizes every month!**

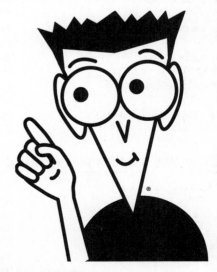

* **Separate Canadian edition also available**

† **Separate U.K. edition also available**

Available wherever books are sold. For more information or to order direct: U.S. customers visit www.dummies.com or call 1-877-762-2974.
U.K. customers visit www.wileyeurope.com or call (0) 1243 843291. Canadian customers visit www.wiley.ca or call 1-800-567-4797.

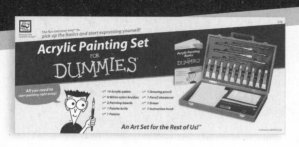
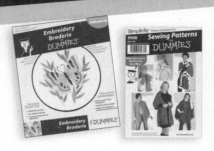
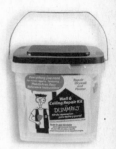
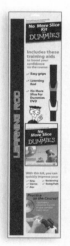
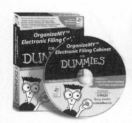
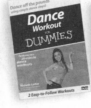

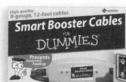
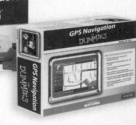
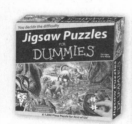
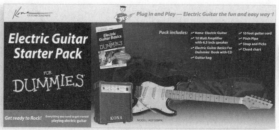
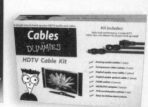
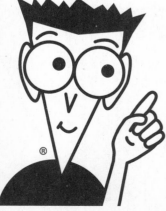

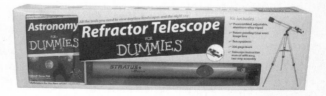
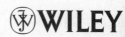